VOCATIONAL AND PERSONAL ADJUSTMENTS IN PRACTICAL NURSING

BETTY GLORE BECKER, R.N., B.S.

Staff Nurse, Our Lady of Victories;
formerly Assistant Director of Nurses, St. Louis County Hospital;
Instructor, Community School of Practical Nursing,
St. Louis–Little Rock Hospital;
Day Surgical Supervisor, St. Louis–Little Rock Hospital;
Head Nurse, Missouri Pacific Hospital;
Assistant Head Nurse, Missouri Pacific Hospital;
Staff Nurse, Missouri Pacific Hospital, St. Louis, Missouri

DOLORES T. FENDLER, R.N., B.S.N., M.Ed.

Formerly Director of School of Practical Nursing, St. Mary's Health Center;
Assistant Director and Surgical Instructor,
School of Practical Nursing, St. Mary's Health Center;
Group Nurse, St. Mary's Health Center and Deaconess Hospital;
Staff Nurse, Surgical Intensive Care Unit,
St. Mary's Health Center, St. Louis, Missouri;
Staff Nurse, Obstetrical Unit, Mercy Hospital,
San Diego, California

SIXTH EDITION

with **16** *illustrations*

The C. V. Mosby Company

ST. LOUIS · BALTIMORE · PHILADELPHIA · TORONTO   1990

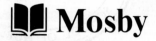 **Mosby**

Editor: Linda L. Duncan
Editorial assistant: Linda Stagg
Production editor: Shauna Burnett Sticht
Book and cover design: Gail Morey Hudson

SIXTH EDITION

Previous editions copyrighted 1970, 1974, 1978, 1982, 1986

Printed in the United States of America

The C.V. Mosby Company
11830 Westline Industrial Drive, St. Louis, Missouri 63146

Library of Congress Cataloging-in-Publication Data

Becker, Betty Glore.
   Vocational and personal adjustments in practical nursing / Betty
Glore Becker, Dolores T. Fendler ; with chapters on ethical and
legal aspects by Laura J. Reilly and leadership and the practical
nurse by Gloria E. Wold. — 6th ed.
       p.   cm.
   Includes bibliographical references.
   ISBN 0-8016-0393-5
   1. Practical nursing.   2. Student adjustment.   3.   Practical
nursing—Vocational guidance.   I.   Fendler, Dolores T., 1922-
II.   Title.
   [DNLM: 1. Nursing, Practical.   WY 195 B395v]
RT62.B43   1990
610.73′069′3 — dc20
DNLM/DLC
for Library of Congress   89-12830
ISBN 0-8016-0393-5   CIP

VT/D/D   9   8   7   6   5   4   3   2   1

Contributors

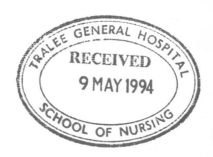

LAURA J. REILLY, R.N., J.D.
Denver, Colorado

GLORIA E. WOLD, R.N., B.S.N., M.S.
Instructor/Lab Manager
Milwaukee Area Technical College
Milwaukee, Wisconsin

To the Instructor

This book has been compiled to assist you in helping students make the necessary professional and personal adjustments inherent in their development as practical nurses. The informal style is designed to capture student interest and enliven factual material to facilitate understanding and retention. We have attempted to pinpoint student ideas and feelings in stated situations; to offer positive suggestions for initiating changes when necessary; to provide basic principles needed for physical, psychological, social, and religious interactions and behavior; to outline systematic plans to implement these principles; and to provide organizational structures and functions that affect and involve practical nurses.

Our expectation in providing you with this book is that it will be a helpful resource in accomplishing your instructional goals. However, it is valueless if you do not have a clear understanding of nursing, of current knowledge of the functions and changes initiated by advances in technology, of societal needs and projects, of the importance and role of the practical nurse as a member of the health team, and of the opportunities available for advancement of practical nurses. Students will look to you for more complete knowledge and practical application of principles described in this book. Unless you can demonstrate that you are a "living image" of these principles, students will be slow to grasp and incorporate them into their personal and professional lifestyles. No book can be a substitute for the *real* you as seen in the ever-watchful eyes of your students.

The terms *practical* and *vocational* nurse are used synonymously in this book. Because the majority of states use the term *practical,* we have generally followed this practice. The practical nurse is referred to as "she," but we recognize the male nurses in the profession. We have attempted to show the relationship between familiar animate and inanimate objects with less tangible traits and characteristics. These relationships should further students' learning abilities and powers to transfer knowledge into meaningful expressions. If knowledge has true meaning for students, they will grasp, retain, and use it in their developmental process.

As with previous editions, we have made an effort to identify and clarify those issues and trends in the health care system that affect practical nursing.

New to this edition are sections on the care of AIDS patients, some advantages and disadvantages of practicing in home health and the hospice unit, and revisions throughout the chapters, including a new chapter on leadership and the practical nurse. We believe these issues to be of vital concern to all health care professionals but of particular relevance to the practice and future of practical nursing.

Visually realistic photographs and artwork have been selected to illustrate situations as they are today in the health care world.

It is our hope that this book will assist you in making your course interesting, alive, and valuable to your students.

We express our sincere appreciation for the interest, encouragement, and assistance we have received from Dolores' husband, Kermit F. Fendler, graduates of St. Mary's Health Center and the Community School of Practical Nursing, and family and friends.

Betty Glore Becker
Dolores T. Fendler

To the Student

The purpose of this book is to help you to understand yourself, to develop your traits to their fullest potential, and to alter and rechannel your less desirable characteristics. The book provides you with positive suggestions for needed change, supplies guidelines for personal and professional behavior and activities, and establishes the necessary requisites inherent in your profession as a practical nurse. It discloses opportunities, organizational structures, and commitments in which you are or will be involved.

In writing this sixth edition, we have tried to incorporate the constructive suggestions and comments of many readers and reviewers so that the book will be more helpful.

Because the profession you have chosen demands knowledgeable practitioners, individual responsibility and specific modes of action are necessary. Through knowledge, awareness, and responsibility, you will be able to develop maturity, which is essential in a practical nurse.

This book is written in an informal style with the hope that you will find the material interesting, informative, and meaningful, thus making it a part of yourself. The practical nurse is referred to as "she," but we recognize the male nurses in the profession. Your future must be founded on a firm, broad foundation if you are to build on it throughout life. The challenge is yours! Your instructors, with the aid of textbooks, can point the way, but they cannot force you to follow given directions. You must choose for yourself. This book will assist you in overcoming obstacles and in making adjustments; it will supply you with knowledge, methods, and principles basic to your profession. By studying the materials and applications, your task will be easier and your adjustment smoother. Remember, this book is only a tool, not an end. If you use it carefully, conscientiously, and with determination, you will succeed in transforming yourself from an untrained student into a skilled licensed practical nurse.

Betty Glore Becker
Dolores T. Fendler

Contents

Appendix C

Appendix D

VOCATIONAL AND PERSONAL ADJUSTMENTS IN PRACTICAL NURSING

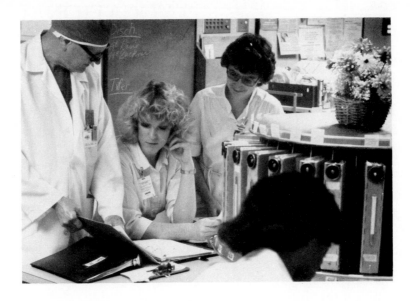

Objectives

At the completion of this chapter the student practical nurse will be able to:

◆ Discuss ways to study smarter, not harder.

◆ Describe the process of communication.

◆ Explain the five steps in problem solving.

1

Practical Nursing as an Educational Program

♦ **The Educational Program**

Some of the days you will long remember are those spent as a practical nurse. You have chosen a career that will present many challenges and require much discipline, a career to serve the best interests of self and society. The following months will be filled with much work and study; however, when you complete the course you will experience a sense of fulfillment and pride in your achievement.

Most schools of practical nursing have an orientation period. The purpose of this period is to familiarize you with the physical facilities and functions of the school so you will feel welcome and comfortable in the environment. During this time the faculty ordinarily reviews the philosophy and objectives of the program and discusses the rules and regulations.

Faculties in schools of practical nursing have a strong commitment to you, the student, and make every effort to assure your success in the program. The practical nursing program is planned to incorporate basic principles with practical experience in a 1-year period. Principles underlying each procedure will precede its practice. It is important for the patient's welfare and for the development of the learning process to know not only *how* to perform a procedure but also *why* you are doing it. The *why* is presented to you in lecture sessions.

Practical nursing programs are designed in various ways to incorporate lecture with practice. Following are some practical nursing programs:

1. Courses in basic principles given in a 16- to 20-week preclinical period with applied practice in the remaining clinical period (32 to 36 weeks); advanced courses given concurrently with specific clinical areas.
2. Courses in basic and advanced concepts given concurrently with practical application during each rotation in clinical areas.

3. Lectures given at a junior college with clinical practice in affiliated institutions (for example, hospitals, nursing homes, and community health programs). Basic courses may be given during a preclinical period or combined with advanced principles during specific clinical rotations.
4. Theory given in a vocational technical school with clinical practice in affiliated institutions. The program of instruction is the same as that in junior colleges.

Basic curriculum includes communications, body structure and function, pharmacology, solutions and dosages, professional adjustments, fundamentals of nursing, mental health, geriatrics, and nutrition and diet therapy; these studies can be applied to all clinical areas. Advanced instruction includes scientific principles, nursing skills, and procedures specific to a clinical area such as obstetrics, psychiatry, or medical-surgical nursing.

◆ Adjustments to Student Life

In addition to the instructional program, student life requires making adjustments to school rules and regulations, to a hospital–medical center environment, to the personalities of various members of the medical team, patients, and family members, and to all the drama, trauma, joy, and sorrow found in a hospital.

Student Counseling

In most schools of practical nursing, faculty members counsel students to ensure academic and professional success. These may be scheduled sessions on a biweekly or bimonthly basis, on an individual basis at the discretion of the faculty member, or from a personal request of the student. Faculty members may direct a student to a professional counselor, often assisting with arrangements, giving encouragement, and communicating with the counselor so the student may obtain the needed guidance.

Study Habits

The following suggestions may help you to study smarter, not harder.

Study ahead of time. Avoid waiting until the day before the test to study. Through study, you will understand the information and be better prepared to take the test. Use the day before the test to review.

Avoid distractions. Close doors to diminish noise. Before you begin to study, tend to your physical needs.

Gather materials. Have available sharp pencils, a dictionary, books, notebook, eraser, and colored marker for highlighting important phrases, ideas, and principles you want to remember.

Reward yourself. Reward yourself only after you have completed the task.

Be confident. Believe that you can and will learn the material.

Scan. Scan the unit or chapter you are about to read. Ask yourself the following questions:

1. What is the chapter all about?
2. What are the main sections of the chapter?
3. Is there a word glossary?
4. Are there questions at the end of the chapter?
5. What do the graphs and illustrations indicate?

Measure. After scanning the chapter, make an assessment of the amount of work and material involved. Be realistic. If there is more material than you can finish in one study session, set a definite time for a second study session.

Look ahead. Read each heading. Understand information given and make up questions you will answer later.

Read and review. Read one section at a time and answer the questions you formulated. Review all the information in one section and be certain you understand the information before proceeding to the next section.

Trace. Examine what you have read. Do you remember the major heading? Are you able to answer the questions at the end of the chapter or unit? Can you define words in the glossary? Are there portions of the chapter you need to review? If so, review and understand before you go on. This technique can also be used as a study review the night before a test.

Take notes. Use *color coding,* yellow or green for highlighting, red for very important items. Use *flip words*. These are words written on corners or insides of pages that call your attention to important phrases or statements. Use *abbreviations;* however, be sure you understand what the abbreviations mean. Use *main headings*. Write notes beneath headings in outline form. Do not write down information you already know. Use complete sentences wherever necessary. *Review* your notes as soon as possible. Remember, much of what is forgotten is forgotten within 24 hours after having been read or heard.

◆ Communication Skills

To communicate, ideas need to travel between the sender and the receiver. The sender is the speaker or writer, the receiver is the listener or the reader. If communication is to be productive, the receiver must comprehend the message the sender is trying to convey.

We must communicate to survive. People depend on other people to meet many of their physiological needs, such as food, water, shelter, and clothing; their environmental needs, such as electricity, cars, and telephones; their emotional needs, such as feeling secure, belonging, and being somebody. Think of what it would be like if we had no automobiles, no clean water, no electricity, no hospitals. The idea is difficult to conceive because we have become accustomed to these comforts. We forget that these comforts originated with someone's ideas and that many people worked together to make them realities.

The ability or inability to communicate affects our relationships with people. Language and communication are interrelated. Try thinking about what you will wear to a party this weekend. Your thoughts entailed words, didn't they?

If someone speaks to you, the sounds become words and you mentally entertain certain ideas. The sender changes these ideas into words and the receiver changes these words back into ideas. If the sender's message matches the idea of the receiver, communication takes place. If not, a breakdown in communication occurs.

Through language, humans are able to express themselves and satisfy their needs and desires. Through communication, people are able to live, work, and play together. The art of communication involves the use of taste, touch, smell, sight, and hearing; in many cases several of these are used simultaneously. For instance, imagine being complimented verbally on your appearance by a person whose eyes tell you he does not mean what he is saying. In such a case you have received two conflicting messages, one verbal and the other nonverbal. You exercise both intelligence and experience to find out exactly what was being communicated. Have you ever found yourself sitting on the edge of your chair after telling someone that you were not in a hurry? This unconscious gesture communicates your real feelings more clearly than words. Have you ever caught yourself handling patients not quite as gently as you should because you disliked them, your supervisor, or yourself? There is something soothing about the touch of a human hand to people who are ill. The pressure applied should be smooth and gentle. If you are overly brisk, believing it to be a sign of efficiency, you impress no one; and your brisk, hasty, and agitated manner will communicate to your patient and others your impatience and lack of caring. Watch carefully that your verbal and nonverbal messages do not contradict each other, because when they do, the nonverbal are the messages people will believe.

Various factors may cause ineffective communication between you and your patient. If you state personal opinions, jump to conclusions, give inappropriate reassurance, change the subject, belittle the patient's feelings, or disapprove or disagree with him, communication is impaired. To develop effective techniques, you must be able to evaluate the individual situation and recognize the need to be observant and objective. Experience, time, and the assistance of your instructors will help you develop these techniques.

In nursing practice the importance of observation is constantly stressed because it enables nurses to be more sensitive "receivers" of nonverbal communication from their patients. In our society it has become an established norm to suppress as much as possible any show of emotion; therefore you find that patients may hesitate to tell you verbally about their fears, worries, or physical discomforts. But as an alert nurse you find they will communicate to you by nonverbal messages. For example, patients may communicate physical discomfort by facial expressions, agitation by restlessness, or fear by crying.

Being a good listener is required of every nurse. Listening is one part of observation. It is also important in developing complete confidence between nurse and patient, an essential therapeutic measure.

There is a difference between hearing and listening. *Hearing* is being in the range of and receiving sound waves, whereas *listening* is the interpretation of spoken words; therefore listening demands a conscious effort on your part. If you really listen to patients, you will listen carefully to things they refrain from saying, as well as to everything they say.

Listening well enables the patient to release emotional tension because talking is an active process. Encouraging patients to talk does not entitle you to probe into their personal lives. Be patient and receptive but remember your role. Once patients suspect you of "invading" their thoughts, they probably will discontinue all communication with you.

Remember that listening to a patient is not the same as social conversation. When the patient tells of some significant experience, you should not relate a similar one of your own. Listen quietly, and practice concentrating on what is said. If you need to express agreement, smile, nod your head, and respond to the cues, but do not interrupt. You may indicate to the patient that you have listened by asking questions or paraphrasing, but never probe.

If you listen carefully, you can discover what people need, what they want, how they feel, and often what they are. Because every patient's situation is different, very little advice can be included on *what* to say. The following suggestions for *how* you speak to a patient may be helpful.

As a health provider it is essential that you acquire an appropriate vocabulary. This helps to avoid the use of wrong words, the omission of important ideas, and the use of long, rambling descriptions that often confuse rather than enlighten a patient. Learn to offer precise, accurate descriptions. Use words sparingly but wisely when communicating with patients or other health professionals. Use your own words to explain technical points to your patients in a simple manner. Speak clearly. A very important sentence loses its meaning when poorly articulated or spoken too quickly or too softly. Many patients are too embarrassed to ask the nurse to repeat an instruction, so they try to decipher what they think they have heard. This can cause a patient needless anxiety and result in unconventional behavior.

The quality of your voice is determined by your vocal cords, but your personality gives your voice an individuality that sets it apart from everyone else's. Words convey only one half of the message; other variants, such as rhythm, stress, timing, tone, pause, pitch, and inflection communicate subtler meanings. Because your voice tells much about you, concentrate on achieving control over it. Practice the art of communication with your classmates.

It is important to organize your thoughts before addressing or answering a patient's questions. A health professional confuses a patient by jumping from one topic to another, interjecting last-minute ideas, and neglecting to either summarize or ask the patient to put into his own words what the nurse has said. Present a caring attitude. The attitude or feeling you express in your spoken interaction with your patient helps communicate genuine concern. Avoid saying the same thing to all patients because they will sense that it is a memorized speech.

Verbal communication with members of the health team should be professional and exclude gossip and confidential information learned while caring for the patient, unless the co-worker has a right to this information.

Written communication is frequently more important than verbal communication because of its far-reaching effects. It is often more accurate and thorough because it requires considerable thought, time, and energy. It also has greater legal implications. Any written communication on a patient's chart can be used not only to inform other members of the health team concerning the patient's progress but also as legal evidence in a court of law. Because the chart is a legal document, it can be used for or against you and the patient. This aspect alone warrants careful, thoughtful charting. Written communication is an effective means of communication, but it can be dangerous if not learned and performed properly.

◆ Problem Solving

Life is full of problem situations, and the nursing profession is no exception. In your daily activities as a student practical nurse, you are faced with many problems. A *problem* can be defined as a lack of balance between the actual and the desired outcome that is of importance to people at a specific time and necessitates an improvement or solution.

You can become frustrated with problems or solve them, thus diminishing stress on yourself and others. Problem solving can become an easier process if you choose a systematic approach.

The following approach may be helpful:

1. *Determine whether you have a problem.* To do this, ask yourself these questions:
   Why do I think I have a problem?
   What would happen if I did nothing about the problem?
   Why am I displeased or dissatisfied?
   If you determine that you have a problem, consider whether it is important enough to warrant further consideration. If not, ignore it. If so, proceed with the next series of steps.
2. *Determine the cause of the problem.*
   Gather together all pertinent data.
   Obtain facts from others and list the information gathered.
   Be objective and do not show partiality to any one person or group of facts.
   Examine the data and determine the cause of the problem.
   You may discover that the cause is a lack of knowledge, communication, a specific skill, poor working relationships, or personality conflicts or that the issue has little meaning to the involved person.
3. *Outline possible solutions to the problem.* By listing specific causes you can determine possible solutions for each cause. Following are examples:
   If the cause is lack of knowledge, consider systematic practice or education.
   If the cause is punishing or nonrewarding consequences to the individual, provide favorable consequences and reduce or eliminate the negative effects.
   If the problem is the result of obstacles that prohibit performance, remove the obstacles.
   A person performs or acts in a certain manner because it has value for him.

Determine the value that a particular action has for this person before trying to develop a workable solution.

4. *Choose and implement the best solution or solutions.*

   Study the possible solutions that you have determined.

   Do not rush to a solution before you have considered all elements of the problem.

   In most situations you will be dealing with infinitely variable entities—human beings—and although probably no perfect solution exists, some solutions are superior to others, and these are the solutions that should be chosen.

   Concentrate on solutions directly related to the problem and choose from these.

   Compare the size of the remedy (solution) to the size of the problem.

5. *Evaluate results.* After implementing the selected solution, be prepared to accept the consequences, good or bad. Evaluate results in terms of the following:

   Was the solution effective? Did it solve the problem satisfactorily?

   What were the shortcomings?

   Could the problem have been solved more satisfactorily through the use of a different solution?

Although problem solving appears to be a long, drawn-out procedure, it can be accomplished in a relatively short time. The process is sensible and not too difficult. It requires you to thoroughly and clearly analyze difficult situations, called *problems*.

Student life is filled with adjustments, problems, interaction, responsibility, communication, study, and involvement. Each of these avenues can assist you in your personal and professional development. A systematic approach to problem solving can aid you in knowing yourself better and in understanding your reactions to fears and problem situations. If you apply yourself earnestly in the beginning of the program, adjustments and solutions can be made more easily and satisfactorily as you progress in your professional and personal career.

◆ *Study Helps*

1. Explain several methods used by practical nursing programs to incorporate theory with clinical practice.
2. List five good study habits.
3. Explain the process of communication.
4. List the three types of communication skills and briefly explain the purpose of each.
5. List and explain the five steps in problem solving.

Bibliography

Collins M: Communication in health care, ed 2, St Louis, 1983, The CV Mosby Co.

King M, Novik L, and Citrenbaum C: Irresistible communication: creative skills for the health professional, ed 1, Philadelphia, 1983, WB Saunders Co.

Milliken ME and Campbell G: Essential competencies for patient care, ed 1, St Louis, 1984, The CV Mosby Co.

Muldary TW: Interpersonal relations for health professionals: a social skills approach, ed 1, New York, 1983, Macmillan Co.

Potter PA and Perry AG: Basic nursing: theory and practice, St Louis, 1987, The CV Mosby Co.

Wrobel-Vaugh BC and Henderson BS: The problem-oriented system in nursing, ed 2, St Louis, 1982, The CV Mosby Co.

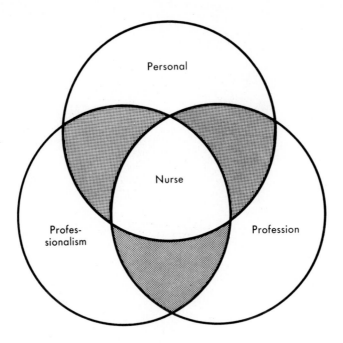

Objectives

At the completion of this chapter the student practical nurse will be able to:

◆ Differentiate between profession and professionalism.

◆ Describe five types of posture.

◆ List five commonly abused drugs, their signs, and their effects.

◆ Discuss health habits essential to the practical nurse.

◆ Discuss personal and professional standards.

The Three P's: the Profession, Professionalism, the Person

◆ Profession Versus Professionalism

A *profession* is defined as an occupation to which one devotes oneself and in which one has specialized expertise. The question is often asked, "Is nursing a profession?" It is generally agreed that for professional status to exist, a profession must have the following:

1. A strong theory base
2. A strong service orientation
3. A code of ethics that is enforced
4. A professional organization that ensures quality of practice
5. Ongoing research
6. An educational standard for all levels of practice

Education increases understanding, awareness, and knowledge. If education is the basis of professionalism and if it is the intent of education to enable individuals to exhibit changed behavior and to make decisions based on their acquired knowledge, then the professional is an individual who follows a line of conduct that reflects these attributes.

All nurses devote themselves to the profession of caring. They have a profound concern for the welfare of others, in particular those who suffer from illness or pain, and it is the qualitative, not the quantitative, elements of this concern that determine whether or not the nurse is a professional.

Practical nursing is the entry level into nursing. The educational program lasts 10 to 12 months. On completion of the program the practical nurse is a skilled and knowledgeable technician. The practical nurse works primarily at the bedside of the patient and under the supervision of the registered nurse. The practical nurse renders safe and quality nursing care.

Nurses play a role, as do all individuals in life, and this role often makes them models for all to see and perhaps imitate. The role requires following a line of conduct. Appearance, behavior, and manners of the professional person should attest to this role.

The student practical nurse has in all probability been taught the importance of appearance, behavior, and manners, and it is not our intent to teach the student these principles but to remind him of their importance when entering the arena of professional practice.

◆ The Person

Appearance

The appearance of the practical nurse should communicate a message of pride in oneself. To do this the nurse must be clean, neatly dressed, and have good posture. A clean nurse is free of body odor. Hair is combed, neatly styled, and washed. Hands and fingernails are especially important. Skin should be smooth, nails short. Excessive makeup, as well as excessive jewelry, is inappropriate to the nurse in uniform. Patients will feel more comfortable with the nurse who looks good.

Posture

What is your opinion of a nurse who displays poor posture? Good posture means the ability to carry oneself well and in correct alignment. This implies shoulders back, chest forward, and abdomen held firm. An exaggerated hip swing may draw attention, and does not promote good body alignment. With the exaggerated hip swing, the sacroiliac and tailbone fail to remain in straight alignment and may cause orthopedic complications in the future. The vertebrae are fitted into each other to allow for bending, lifting, and stooping, but undue pressure at any one point may cause strain and ensuing pain.

One of the courses you will encounter in training is body mechanics. It teaches you how to move, bend, and stoop. Correct weight bearing and balance of the body are very important to the nurse to prevent physical disability. Walking straight with shoulders back, sitting erect with the back resting against the back of the chair and the feet placed flat on the floor, and stooping with the knees bent are ways of maintaining good body alignment throughout the day, not only in your busy professional life but also in your personal life.

Posture indicates how we feel about ourselves. Different postures are associated with varying emotional states. We usually think the person with an erect posture and squared shoulders is self-confident and capable. The person walking with shoulders bowed, head thrust forward, and eyes looking down communicates a lack of self-confidence and symbolizes a person carrying a heavy burden. An individual standing erect with hands on hips appears autocratic and dominant. Someone sitting with arms folded and shoulders curled inward portrays resignation and abandonment. A relaxed posture is a good indicator of feeling and status. Relaxed postures are evident in individuals having a conversation in which they share similar views. When you are with another person your posture reflects your attitude toward that person. For this reason nurses must be particularly careful of the way they stand at the bedside of a patient. If their attitude is one of caring, their posture should be erect, not rigid; relaxed, not slouched; positive, not submissive. The qualities of your personal life need to be carried over into your professional life and vice versa. You cannot regard yourself as a desk with drawers, one drawer for your professional life and the other your personal life, constructed in such a manner that one drawer can be opened and the other closed. These two aspects of your life are interrelated; they affect and depend on each other.

Health

Diet. Nurses must eat a regular and balanced diet to function properly, to keep physically fit, and to set an example for others. Nursing students are frequently diet offenders. They skip meals, eat improperly balanced diets, and follow crash diets. Students who skip breakfast for 10 minutes of extra sleep cannot function well. By midmorning they are frequently weak from hunger and unable to think correctly, thereby decreasing efficiency. This is a harmful practice. A good breakfast is a must if you are to perform nursing duties correctly and intelligently. Proper foods provide the nutrients and energy to carry out these activities.

The four basic food groups provide the foundation for selection of all nutrients required by the normal adult. The National Research Council formulated and published the following recommended daily allowances for normal American adults from each of the four food groups: dairy products—two or more cups of milk or its equivalent; meat group (meat, fish, eggs, and poultry)—two or more servings daily; vegetables and fruits—four or more servings daily; breads and cereals—four or more servings daily. The Council planned the Recommended Daily Allowances (RDA) to provide a margin of safety in the specified allowances to ensure maximum nutritional intake. Developing intelligent food habits founded on the basic four food groups and the RDA is one of the keys to your success as a student and as a licensed practical nurse.

To lose weight your calorie intake must be less than the amount lost in normal energy. Reduction may occur as the result of eating balanced, nutritional meals in place of high-calorie meals. A regular exercise routine will also help to burn unwanted calories. Remember to consult a physician before starting a strict reduction diet or exercise routine.

Rest and sleep. Everyone needs sufficient rest and sleep to do a job well. The amount of sleep may vary with the individual. An infant or child requires more sleep than the young or middle-aged adult, who may need only 6 to 8 hours of sleep. Individual need is the determining factor of the amount of sleep required. Do not compare yourself with others. You may have a friend who requires only 5 hours of sleep. With this amount he can function without stress or strain. If you were to limit yourself to 5 hours of sleep when you need 8, this need would quickly manifest itself in your daily activities. You might show signs of fatigue, irritability, and lack of ambition. Your resistance to infections would be lessened. As a result you might suffer frequent colds, flu, or serious infections.

Sleep is a natural process and essential to restore body powers. During the hours of sleep body parts are at their lowest ebb of functioning. They appear to be at a complete stage of rest or inactivity; however, complete inactivity cannot take place because body functions must continue in order to maintain life.

Rest is as important as sleep. Rest means the conscious freedom from activity. This rest can be mental, physical, or both. Physical rest means minimal activity of the body. Mental rest means minimal activity of the mind. If you are relaxed and are at peace with yourself, you are in a state of mental rest. There is no turmoil churning about in your mind. Rest requires the combination of both physical and mental processes.

Alcohol. Many of you may be in the age group that is permitted the use of alcohol. Socially, alcohol consumption in moderation can increase interpersonal relationships between friends and acquaintances by producing a relaxed state in many individuals. It may allay tensions and anxieties.

Its abuse, however, is always detrimental physically and emotionally. In our rapidly changing society alcoholism is increasing. It can no longer be viewed as a moral issue. It is an illness.

Initially alcohol produces a feeling of well-being; latently it acts on the brain and spinal cord as a nervous system depressant. Alcoholism may lead to confusion, stupor, and mental and physical deterioration, depending on the amount and length of consumption. Persons addicted to alcohol are seldom cured without the willpower to abstain completely from its use. One drink initiates the compulsive desire for more. Alcoholism plays an important part in crimes, accidents, the need for medical care, and industrial losses by causing decreased production and increased absenteeism.

Drugs. Drugs should be taken only when prescribed by and under the supervision of a physician. As a nurse you have the obligation to give only those drugs ordered by a physician. Under no condition may you make any drug available to another person without the written order of the physician.

Drug addiction is a serious problem today. It is the result of drug abuse, lack of information, "innocent" experimentation, and the need for group identity. Scarcely a day passes that one does not read or hear about tragedies caused by drug abuse: overdoses, "bad trips," addiction, suicide, and crime. As a nurse you must not only refrain from drug abuse but also have facts and be able to recognize the common signs of abuse in others (Table 1).

Commonly used addicting drugs that are available in most hospitals include narcotics such as morphine, meperidine, hydrochloride (Demerol), dihydromorphinone (Dilaudid), and barbiturates.

Drug abuse depends on the amount and strength of the dose, the purity of the drug, and the user's surroundings, mood, emotional stability, and unique body chemistry.

Smoking. Smoking should never be done in a patient's room. Smoking in unauthorized places can be a fire hazard, and great care should be taken to enforce the safety rules of the institution for patients and visitors. It has been scientifically proven that smoking can have harmful physical effects by interfering with oxygen intake.

◆ Mental Health Habits

Mental health is something positive: peace of mind, happiness, and enjoyment and satisfaction from a job well done. It comes with the satisfactory adjustment of your desires, ambitions, ideals, and feelings to the daily demands of living. Ordinarily a mentally healthy person feels comfortable with himself and others and is able to cope effectively with the demands of society. This includes the development of an open but analytical mind and shunning gossip and backbiting. Strive to see the good in others; stress good qualities when found, rather than those less desirable. Help to develop friendships, and uphold your friends and their reputations. As this type of nurse, you will be appreciated for your integrity and character.

Basic Needs

From childhood you have learned the basic needs of all humans: affection, success, and security. The manner in which each of these needs is met depends on the individual. People need to be loved and accepted by others. You may require more love than others, depending on your individual personality; however, you must give love before you can receive it. As a social being, directly or indirectly responsible for the happiness of others, you are compelled to give this love to others. A person who loves is a generous, selfless person and thinks about another's welfare before his own. This type of person, although not expecting or demanding a return of this love, cannot help but receive love or respect in return for generosity. This is the cherished friend, the one on whom you can depend to give you a helping hand. A friend is a person you love and respect. In giving love, you receive love in return.

As a student you need the respect of your fellow students, instructors, patients, members of the medical team (although it may take time to establish this relationship), and other hospital personnel. You want to be accepted and to feel as though you are a part of each of these groups. Only in true acceptance can you find happiness in your profession. You can encourage this acceptance by learning and developing the qualifications, techniques, and skills that are essential in both your professional and personal life.

Almost everyone wants success and achievement. Because there are degrees of achievement, there must be involved effort, perseverance, and challenge. The degree of accomplishment depends on the individual. Success in nursing depends on your efforts to study and learn about your profession and apply these facts in practical situations. Because this process will be full of trials and challenges, you must persevere in your efforts. If nursing had not presented a challenge to you, you would have sought another profession. A challenge spurs you to attempt to attain something that is "out of your reach" at the present time. The challenge is strengthened by your determination and your ideas. If you want to become a good nurse, you must not allow anything to interfere with your desire and goal.

Table 1 ◇ Most commonly abused drugs today

Drug	Action	Signs	Effects
Stimulants			
Oral amphetamines (pep and diet pills) "Bennies" "Dexies" "Uppers"	Stimulates central nervous system	Overactive Talkative Lack of appetite Dependence on drug	Confusion Unpredictable, irrational, and violent behavior Fatigue Decreased bodily resistance to illness
Injectable amphetamines "Speed" "Meth"	Fast acting Increases heart rate Increases blood pressure	Confusion Extreme fatigue Depression Mood swings	Violent behavior Toxic psychosis May cause shock and death
Cocaine/"crack" "Big C" "Blow" "Burese" "Carrie" "Coke" "Gold dust" "Nose powder" "Snowbird" "Superblow" "White girl" "Rock" "Base"	Stimulates central nervous system	Increases psychic energy Feelings of self-confidence Intense sexuality Excitability Euphoria Anxiety Feeling of well-being followed by depression Delusions Irritability Sleeplessness	Increased heart beat, blood pressure, and pulse Dilated pupils Nausea and vomiting Occasional hallucinations Confusion Insomnia Impotence Addiction Seizures Severe depression Paranoia Lung damage Heart attack Sudden death
Depressants			
Barbiturates Secobarbital (Seconal) Pentobarbital (Nembutal) Secobarbital and amobarbital (Tuinal)	Depresses central nervous system	Drowsiness Slurred speech Depression Deep sleep	Mental and physical dependence Depression Slurred speech Coma and possible death

Drug	Action	Signs	Effects
Heroin "Big H" "Horse" "Junk" "Stuff" "Black Tar"	Depresses central nervous system	Pinpoint pupils Needle tracks Craving for sweets and liquids Dreamlike disposition Aggressive or violent behavior when in need of "fix" Psychological dependence on drug Pallid complexion Boils at site of injections	Physical addiction Need of increased dose regularly Withdrawal pains Psychological dependence Can cause hepatitis, septicemia, and infection of heart valves Infection of bloodstream, heart, and lungs Blood clots in lungs Possible death
Methaqualone "Quas" "Sopes" "Quads"	Depresses central nervous system	Slurred speech Disorientation Drunken behavior	Shallow respirations Mental and physical dependence Depression Coma and possible death

Hallucinogens

Drug	Action	Signs	Effects
LSD "Acid" "Beast" "Sugar" "Coffee"	Injures and alters central nervous system and brain tissue	Irrational behavior Panic Disorganized mind	Auditory and visual hallucinations Bizarre behavior Chromosome changes Birth defects Depersonalization Psychosis
Marijuana "Grass" "Pot" "Weed" "Mary Jane" "Reefer"	Injures and alters central nervous system and brain tissue	Dilated pupils Bloodshot eyes Sensitivity to light Craving for sweets Mood swings	Releases inhibitions Alters reality Bizarre behavior Distortions of time and space
Phencyclidine "Angel dust" "DOA" "Hog" "PCP"	Veterinary anesthetic Injures and alters central nervous system and brain tissue	Flushing Profuse sweating Analgesia Muscle incoordination Dizziness Nausea Vomiting	Unpleasant experience Visual or auditory hallucinations Preoccupation with death Depersonalization Poor perception of time and distance

If you are a stable individual, you will feel secure. You will not be swayed in any direction. However, this does not mean being stubborn or opinionated. You must know what to do, know how to do it, and have practice and experience in doing it. The more you do something, the more secure you feel in doing it. You must be willing to accept a better way of doing something if a better way becomes apparent even though you may feel less secure at the beginning. In the nursing profession you must know your duties, know how to perform them, and be experienced in performing them.

You cannot help others with problems if you do not recognize that you also have problems. You must know what the problems and their possible solutions are and then choose and carry out the solutions. You need to understand your own reactions to various conditions and people. Only by controlling your feelings are you able to help others. For example, a patient becomes angry because he feels that he is receiving poor or insufficient nursing care. If you are the first person he encounters, he may begin to tell you in no uncertain terms what he thinks about the hospital, his physician, the nursing staff, and perhaps you as an individual. Your reaction, if you are quick-tempered, may be to defend all involved, answering the patient in the same tone of voice that he is using. However, if you know that you have a quick temper, you can take positive steps to control it. In this instance you could count to 10 before you speak and answer the patient kindly and in a soft voice. You may tell him that you are sorry that he feels this way and try to determine what has happened to initiate his response. You may discover that the physician has told him that he has an incurable disease. The patient may not wish to accept this condition and attempts to fight it by finding fault with the hospital, the nursing personnel, and so on. If you become angry, you may never discover the patient's real problem and will fail to help him. You need to know yourself thoroughly to handle the patient's feelings.

Personality

Do you know what makes you different from your fellow students? It is your personality. Personality includes traits, habits, attributes, and physical characteristics, as well as behavioral and emotional tendencies that you specifically manifest. You often hear or say, "Sally certainly has a pleasant personality." By this you mean that Sally has certain tendencies or traits that you find desirable. Personality is a difficult quality to evaluate because it is subjective and dependent on the person evaluating. The evaluator can be influenced by pleasant mannerisms and desirable traits and characteristics. You make yourself into the kind of person you are. If you want to develop a pleasant personality, you must know yourself, love life and people, and care about people and accept them as they are. You must be able to cope with everyday problems that confront you without building up strong tensions and frustrations. A positive outlook enables you to influence those around you, enrich your personality, and make yourself more acceptable to friends and companions without losing your identity.

Mature personality is a state of full growth or maximum development of traits, characteristics, and mannerisms that enables you to act and react in an adult manner to situations, problems, and interpersonal contacts. This state can be acquired through the learning process from personal experiences, knowledge, and interaction with others. It is learned and developed through trial and error, mistakes (yours and others'), physical maturation of body cells, and the educational process.

Charm, Poise, and Dignity

Charm is never artificial; it is part of the person. If you are a delightful person, others want to associate with you and are pleased and happy when you come into their presence.

Poise denotes calmness, evenness of temper, and composure. Much thought and practice are needed to obtain the desired results in this area.

Dignity implies self-control. Dignity and self-control enable you to be efficient in emergency situations and perform your designated tasks while manifesting kindness and empathy.

Tension

Tension is stress or the accumulation of inner pressures. It is caused by conflict of two opposing forces. For example, a woman who is married to an alcoholic husband may try repeatedly to satisfy her husband in every way so that his need for alcohol is diminished. After repeated efforts without success, she may decide to leave him. What are the two opposing forces in this situation? One is the fact that she loves him and wants to help him; she married him for better or worse and wants to fulfill her side of the marriage contract. The other is the fact that he refuses her help; he mistreats her with verbal and physical attacks. Because she believes that she cannot withstand this type of treatment any longer, she decides to leave him. These two forces battle within her. Only one can win; either she remains with her alcoholic husband and suffers the abuse he imposes on her, or she leaves him and is freed from him and his abuses. This battle builds up emotional pressures within her. These pressures may appear in various ways unless she can find a suitable outlet for them. They can develop into physical symptoms such as headaches or pain. They can lead to the creation of a dream world and loss of contact with reality. She may find suitable outlets for these pressures through physical activities such as playing a strenuous game of tennis or actively participating in community organizations and activities.

As a student nurse how can you cope with daily tensions and prevent their accumulation? For example, you are working on a busy nursing unit staffed with one registered nurse, several students, and assistants to care for the entire patient load. This means that your assignment may be too great to accomplish adequately. You can become frustrated in carrying out the assignment, speaking sharply to the patients and your peers and complaining about the lack of help, or you may take a few minutes to plan your work for the morning. You may not be able to give each patient the amount of time that you would like to give, but you can plan to give each patient the amount of care that he needs. In the latter case you are able to accomplish more for all concerned. You remain calm, the work is accomplished to the best of your ability, and good relationships are maintained. By coping effectively with one day's situation, you are better prepared to handle future situations without increasing tensions.

Attitudes

Attitudes—feelings about people, places, and things—can be positive or negative. They are positive if you seek the good in things, if you see life as worth living, and if you see it as something good and challenging. Life has been given to you to use, enjoy, and cherish. You must love people and think kindly of them. Your friends and peers have faults, as you do, but their good qualities far exceed their less desirable characteristics. You have to believe that some things happen for good. Evil exists because there is a lack of goodness, but it gives you the opportunity to profit from another's mistakes as well as your own.

Negative attitudes stifle your growth. They are like a stone tied to your neck. They prevent you from accomplishing things that you want to achieve. They make you sullen and lonely, because the negative person has few friends.

Habits

Habit is the acquired consistent repetition of behavior. It is something that you do over and over until you do it unconsciously. For example, you may have the habit of brushing your teeth each morning after breakfast. By the repetition of this act you have trained yourself to the point that the act becomes automatic. You immediately brush your teeth after breakfast without giving much thought to the process. This is a good habit because it helps keep your mouth fresh and odorless and eliminates bacteria harbored around the teeth and gums.

You may also have the acquired habit of chewing on your fingernails when you become tense. This is a poor habit because it not only looks unprofessional but also may cause infection. Bacteria may become embedded under the nails, and while you are chewing on your nails, bacteria may be transferred into the mouth and cause disease.

◆ Standards for Professional and Personal Conduct

To ensure the continuance of institutional harmony and unity, you must be familiar with the institution's structure, organization, administration, services, departments, and accreditation. As a licensed practical nurse working in a hospital or other institutional setting, certain types of behavior or characteristics will be expected of you. These include courtesy, honesty, etiquette, shop talk, telephone manners, dining room manners, enthusiasm, and cooperation. Each of these will be discussed separately.

Courtesy

Courtesy is a polite act or remark. It is necessary in establishing satisfactory group relationships. In everyday life common courtesies should be shown to friends and neighbors. As a nurse you must manifest courtesy when dealing with patients, relatives, co-workers, and other members of the health team. Politeness is comparable to the "shine on the apple." It gives the "finishing touch" to a person and generates acceptance from others.

Courtesy can be shown in many ways. A sincere, cheerful greeting ordinarily elicits a response. Its effect is contagious. Simple expressions of "thank you" and "please" produce wonders in human relationships. Courtesy emphasizes the dignity and respect of one person for another. The most gratifying trait you can develop, if you do not already possess it, is to recognize the achievements of others through words, gestures, or actions.

You will gain the cooperation of your patient by being courteous to him. Indicate that you respect him by addressing him properly, using his correct name, "Mr. Smith" or "Mr. Jones"; refrain from calling him "Pop," "Grandpa," or by his first name. Every patient wants to retain his identity. Another courteous gesture is explaining in advance any procedure you must perform. This explanation alleviates anxiety and indicates to the patient that you care about him as a person.

One important form of courtesy you must remember as a nurse is to knock on a closed door before entering. This may save the patient embarrassment and will secure the privacy to which he has a right. Other forms of politeness include not interrupting a conversation unless absolutely necessary, stepping aside to allow someone in a hurry to pass easily, offering an apology, and excusing yourself when leaving a group. Courtesy is the diamond that can be placed in any setting. It enriches the person and portrays the sparkling qualities so attractive to others.

Honesty

A practical nurse must be a person of high integrity. This implies the faithful adherence to moral and ethical principles that are expected of you as a professional person. The nursing profession trusts you to act in the best interests of the patient. This includes charting treatments and medications accurately, carrying out physicians' orders as written, reporting unintentional errors immediately to the proper authorities, not willfully performing or assisting with any procedure or act detrimental to the patient, and performing only those procedures for which you have been sufficiently prepared.

Honesty and economy work hand in hand. If you are honest with your employer and your patients, you will not be wasteful of time or materials. Wastefulness is costly. It may result in a rise in hospital operating expenses, and ultimately this cost will be reflected on the patient's bill. Wastefulness also may keep your salary at a lower scale.

Time is a costly item to all institutions and businesses. When added together, minutes spent daydreaming, talking about others, and avoiding work amount to large sums of wasted money. Lost time lowers the standards of nursing care.

Careless use of equipment and materials can be costly to the patient and the hospital. Hospital equipment and supplies, because of their delicacy and unique craftsmanship, are expensive items. Thoughtless contamination of sterile equipment may cause harm to your patient and result in infectious processes and financial deficits. You have the obligation to respect the rights of others in all matters that directly or indirectly apply to them. Learn to use time, equipment, and supplies to the best possible advantage.

Etiquette

Etiquette can be defined as a code of accepted behavior. This code includes social graces and manners. It means acceptable or required forms or manners of behavior that should be manifested in specific situations. Rules of etiquette change with the times and vary within different societies. The purpose of these rules is to serve as guidelines to be followed to prevent awkward situations and embarrassment.

All institutions have rules of etiquette. They may be written or traditional. Some hospitals have more rigid performance standards than others. The rules of etiquette in a hospital are similar to those that should be practiced in everyday situations. If doubt arises as to what is proper in the hospital setting, common sense and dignity should solve the problem in most situations; if not, seek the advice of the nursing service director, head nurse, supervisor, personnel director, or in-service coordinator.

When making introductions, address the person of greater authority and introduce the person of lesser authority, for example, "Miss Jones (RN), may I introduce Miss Brown (SPN)." Introduce the younger person to the older person in the same manner, for example, "Grandpa, I would like to introduce my friend Jackie to you." If a person has a title, state the title, such as "Dr. Smith, may I introduce Mrs. Tee, our director of nursing service."

Shop Talk

Shop talk is common among employees. It may be defined as a discussion of the various factors of one's work. There is no harm in discussing work itself. However, when it involves names, personalities, and a physician's treatment of a patient, it is unethical. As a result you may be liable to court action for indulging in slander. Do not become too personal! Talk about general things. Do not discuss work in public places, on the bus, in the dining area, or at home. Avoid gossiping about other personnel; it is disloyal and unfair. Take great care in answering questions of relatives, patients, and members of the health team.

Telephone Manners

The telephone is an important means of communication. The following are definite rules regarding its use:
1. Answer in a courteous, friendly tone of voice. This implies the avoidance of a saccharine or curt response. Speak correctly and plainly, neither too rapidly nor too slowly.
2. Identify your location, name, and title. For example, "5 West, Miss Read, practical nurse" immediately conveys to the caller the area reached, the person speaking, and her position. If the call is for someone else, this saves time for you and the caller.
3. Summon the proper person to the phone or record the message. If the person is not available, ask the caller if there is a message or if he prefers to call later when the person is available.
4. All calls made on duty should be brief, courteous, accurate, and necessary.
5. Never give unauthorized information over the phone. When giving any type of information, know to whom you are speaking.
6. When receiving a call that requires time to gather the needed information, ask the caller if he prefers to hold or have you return the call. Make sure you have the correct number if you are to return the call.
7. Replace the receiver gently. Banging the receiver contributes to poor public relations, does not improve your frame of mind, and is wearing on the instrument.

Hospital telephones are limited to professional calls. Personal calls are referred to the personnel or nursing service departments or to the nursing school office. In cases of emergency these departments will take a message and deliver it to you, or they will transfer the call directly to you.

Dining Room Manners

Mealtime is an occasion for relaxation as well as for eating. Most institutions provide pleasant and cheerful cafeterias for their employees because they realize the effect that mealtime has on employee proficiency. Meals may be paid for by the employer or priced at reasonable rates. Great effort is made to provide employee comfort.

However, it must be the joint effort of everyone eating in the dining area to maintain a relaxing atmosphere. This includes good table manners, avoidance of boisterous talking and laughing, and waiting patiently in cafeteria lines. Table manners should be the same as those used in a restaurant or in your home. They involve the proper use of utensils and refined eating habits. While you are on duty, you should avoid foods that leave odors. These odors may be irritating to patients and co-workers. Good posture should also be maintained. Do nothing to distract others. Mealtime is a rest period that everyone deserves. You have the obligation to help maintain this type of atmosphere.

Enthusiasm and Cooperation

Enthusiasm and cooperation are treasured characteristics. They help build employee morale and create good working conditions and relationships between departments within the institution. In essence they stimulate workers to give their best to the job.

However, enthusiasm should never encroach on the duties of fellow workers. In other words, you should never attempt to assume anyone else's duties. Most institutions have job descriptions stating the specific duties for each job category. Job descriptions define and eliminate overlapping activities among employees. Enthusiasm and cooperation imply helping others and working together with a genuine interest in what each is accomplishing for the patient's welfare.

Enthusiasm and cooperation make the patient feel secure and confident. They enable the patient to feel comfortable and content because he knows all are interested in his recovery and are willing to do everything necessary and requested. A good relationship between the patient and nurse is a valuable tool in the patient's recovery.

◇   ◇   ◇

It is important for you to learn, if you have not already done so, that physical and mental factors greatly influence your personal and professional activities. You must be convinced that life is worth living and live it to the fullest so that you can find happiness in your own life and give happiness to all with whom you come into contact. Because you are a member of the health team, do your job to the best of your ability at all times.

◆ *Study Helps*

1. Define the term *profession*.
2. What changes the behavior of the individual? Give examples.
3. Discuss the importance of good posture.
4. What are the effects of alcoholism?
5. List five drugs commonly abused in our society. State the signs and effects of each drug.
6. Define *habit*. State one good and one bad habit that you have.
7. Define *courtesy* and give examples of its practical applications in the nursing field.
8. How can a practical nurse manifest honesty and economy in nursing?
9. List several rules of etiquette. State your feelings regarding their application.
10. List and explain seven rules for answering the telephone.
11. Explain the effect of enthusiasm and cooperation on the patient.

Bibliography

Carlson R: Issues and trends in health, St Louis, 1987, The CV Mosby Co.

Chenevert M: Special techniques in assertiveness training for women in the health professions, ed 3, St Louis, 1988, The CV Mosby Co.

Davis AJ: Listening and responding, ed 1, St Louis, 1983, The CV Mosby Co.

Harkness G and Dincher JR: Total patient care: foundations and practice, ed 7, St Louis, 1987, The CV Mosby Co.

Jacobson SF and McGrath HM: Nurses under stress, ed 1, New York, 1983, John Wiley & Sons, Inc.

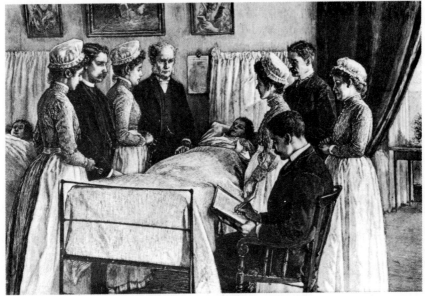

Objectives

At the completion of this chapter the student practical nurse
will be able to:

◆ Describe the development of nursing from ancient times through
the eras to modern day.

◆ Describe the development of practical nursing from its earliest
time through the modern day.

◆ Identify, by name and accomplishment, those who influenced
nursing and practical nursing.

◆ Explain the role of the practical nurse as a member of the
health team.

History and Trends of Professional and Practical Nursing

When you think of history, your thoughts often revert to something that is ancient and dead. However, history is in the making every day. Your actions today will in some way affect the lives of others tomorrow. They serve to pave the road of the nursing profession to greater achievements. Because your actions and activities will have far-reaching effects on the future, you should know the part the past has played in your life today. Nursing dates back to earliest times of mankind.

◆ Nursing in Ancient Civilizations

In ancient times nursing was not a formal occupation based on scientific principles. The development of nursing in history is closely linked with, although not necessarily parallel to, medical history. It is probable that neither medicine nor nursing could have developed without the other. Nursing existed in practice although not in name.

Nursing functions were frequently performed by a member of a sick person's household, a relative, or a servant. Childbirth was accompanied by some type of nursing care of both mother and child by midwives and wet nurses. The temple, a center of religion, was a healing place where nursing functions were performed by a priest, priestess, or deaconess.

As medicine developed scientifically, physicians began to impart their knowledge to students, who were responsible for the care and observation of the patient.

With advancement of the woman's position in society and achievement of educational, economic, and political freedoms, parallel gains were made in nursing. This freedom for women was necessary for nursing to develop as a profession.

Babylonia

In early Mesopotamia sickness was regarded as a punishment for sin, and the ill were cared for within the household by a slave or domestic servant. Historical documents prove that nursing duties such as bathing, bandaging, and massaging the patient were performed in this civilization.

One of the ancient Babylonian kings, Hammurabi, compiled a code of law (2000 BC) that placed legal limitations on those treating the sick. This code was designed as a protective measure for patients.

Egypt

Egyptian medicine contained contrasting elements of mysticism, realism, magic, and empiricism.

Training schools for physicians were attached to many of the temples. There is evidence that one such school existed around 1100 BC. Temple priests were responsible for nursing care functions, such as bathing. Medical students were involved in the care and observation of patients. In addition, lay persons with special knowledge or talents in this area were frequently excused from work to care for the sick.

The best source of knowledge about ancient Egyptian nursing techniques can be found in the *Edwin Smith Surgical Papyrus*, which gives detailed instructions for the daily care of patients.

It may surprise today's nurses to know that their counterparts in ancient Egypt recorded the pulse and used present-day techniques and materials, such as bandages and splints, in the care and treatment of the sick and wounded.

Israel

The Old Testament is an excellent resource on Hebrew history. Many passages refer to wet nurses and those who nursed the sick or acted as companions.*

In the area of medicine the Hebrew priest functioned as a public health officer. Nursing, confined to the home, was rendered by women of the community.

Although the Hebrews borrowed their medical knowledge from the Babylonians and Egyptians, they were unique in that they generously shared this knowledge with succeeding civilizations.

Greece

The Greek woman's lack of freedom limited the progress of nursing because it restricted nursing duties to household members.

However, progress in the field of medicine was monumental and indirectly affected nursing. Hippocrates (460-370 BC) was responsible for this medical progress. He introduced the scientific method in the diagnosis and treatment of patients, which eliminated the mythical and magical elements of treatment. For 2000 years Hippocrates has been known as the Father of Medicine.

His emphasis on close observation, medical and surgical treatment, and care of patients reveals a dependence of physicians on medical students and trained nurses to carry out these functions. The Greeks were the first to become conscious of the need for *trained* nurses.

In Greek society birth was also attended by midwives and nurses. Socrates' mother was a nurse-midwife.

---

*Numbers 11:12; Exodus 2:7, 2:9; II Kings 4:4; Genesis 24:59, 35:8.

Rome

Roman medicine was a product of that civilization's thirst for conquest. Greek physicians who were Roman prisoners of war brought with them Hippocratic medicine. Before this time medicine was a mixture of common sense remedies and superstition.

Although the Romans added little to the field of medicine, they recognized the need for nursing and expanded it into a specialized field. Their conquests were responsible for the establishment of military hospitals with nurse attendants. Roman soldiers were trained in basic first aid techniques. Buildings or rooms on large Roman estates served as hospitals and were staffed by "professional nurses" who were probably slaves.

China

There is no reference in the literature of Ancient China to nurses. If there were nurses they probably were not women, because Confucius defined woman's position as inferior to man. The woman's place was in the home and her greatest value was when she produced a son.

India

Ancient Indian writings from 800 BC to 2 AD set standards and qualifications for male nurses. These included knowledge, preparation and compounding of drugs for administration, devotedness to the patient, cleverness, and purity of body and mind. Technical skills, which included bathing, rubbing and massaging, lifting and moving the patient, and bedmaking, were emphasized. Nurses were to be untiring in their service to the sick.

◆ Nursing in the Early Christian Era (50-476 AD)

About the time of Christ's birth, Rome had reached its supremacy. Christianity was rarely manifested openly because it was prohibited by the emperor. However, as Rome declined, Christianity spread and grew. Organized nursing came into existence as an expression of charity. St. Paul introduced Phoebe of Cenchreae into Rome as a deaconess of the church. One of her duties was to care for the sick. Phoebe is known as the first visiting nurse and the first deaconess in the church. Grasping the spirit of this new Christianity, other Christian convents formed orders to care for the sick and poor.

History records that Fabiola, a wealthy matron, founded a hospital in Rome in atonement for the sin of having a second marriage. She rendered personal care to the sick and injured, and no disease was too grave or too contagious to prevent her from giving care. Her good deeds became known among the elite. In a short time Marcella and Paula, two other wealthy matrons, joined in this charitable work. Nursing progressed until the Dark Ages.

◆ Nursing During the Dark and Middle Ages (476-1450 AD)

Little is known about nursing in the Dark Ages. However, we know that learning of all types was kept alive through the great literary works of that period. Christians, who brought about organized nursing care, were again persecuted, and followers of Christianity hid behind walls of monasteries and convents. Various religions included in their practices not only the conversion of heathens but also the care of the sick. In the medical field hospitals were founded; the most noted were Hôtel-Dieu in Lyons in 542 AD, Hôtel-Dieu in Paris in 650 AD, and Santo Spirito in Rome in 717 AD. Although nursing history during this period remains obscure, it can be assumed, because new hospitals were founded and staffed by trained personnel who enabled them to achieve the fame for which they are known and recorded in history.

The two main factors influencing nursing during the Middle Ages were religion and the military. Because monks and nuns assumed most of the nursing duties, new and additional monasterial orders were founded. A number of these were military orders that trained men in the techniques of fighting and the care of the sick. One such order was the Knights Hospitalers, who were formally approved of by the pope in 1113. Men belonging to this order ministered to their own sick and wounded soldiers, worked in general hospitals rendering the needed nursing care, and fought in defense of the reigning political power. Two additional military orders, the Knights Templars and Teutonic Knights, came into existence. All performed similar duties and received uniform training. As time progressed, the religious duty of caring for the sick predominated over the military duty. This is not surprising in view of the fact that the primary concern of established religious orders was the care of the sick and poor.

During the Middle Ages cleanliness and ventilation as known today were nonexistent. Buildings were constructed with windows too high to open. There were few, if any, facilities for plumbing, heating, and lighting. In many instances linens had to be carried to and washed in the river. Nursing care was primitive and consisted chiefly of administering medications, bathing patients, dressing wounds, and providing for the physical needs of patients.

Accustomed as we are in the United States to the latest conveniences in hospital construction, facilities, and equipment, we would consider medical facilities and nursing care in the Middle Ages crude and deficient. However, similar conditions exist today in poverty-stricken and underdeveloped nations. In these countries hospitals are constructed without heat, with poor lighting facilities with frequently nonfunctioning electrical power, and with inadequate plumbing to meet patients' needs. Linens are washed in cold water in outdoor concrete sinks and are cleansed by rubbing soiled areas with rough rocks. Inhabitants of such countries wash their clothing in nearby streams and rivers. Nursing remains primitive. Medications are given to the patient only if the family can provide them. Bathing is infrequent because of lack of heat and warm water. The nurse dresses wounds, assists with uncomplicated surgical procedures (complicated procedures are not performed), and attempts to meet the physical needs of patients. Are these not conditions similar to those that existed in the Middle Ages?

During the Middle Ages societal structure changed to include a third, or middle, class of people between the poor and the rich. Several factors united and effected this development. The Christian religion dominated all aspects of the Western World. The church functioned as the head and power of the collective small cities in Europe. Cathedrals and universities were founded. Buying and selling between cities and, later, nations became a common practice. The cultural flow between Europe and the Orient was initiated by those participating in the Crusades. The combination of these factors necessitated the development of a middle class to carry forward these achievements.

Nursing was also affected by the development of the middle class. This can be illustrated by the life and activities of St. Catherine of Siena (1347-1380). Catherine gave herself untiringly to the care of the sick. When the plague came to Siena in 1372, she worked day and night nursing its victims. The greatest problem at this time was the need for some type of transportation of the sick to hospitals. In response to this need Catherine organized the first ambulance service. Today the Hospital at La Scala stands as a memorial to Catherine for her heroic efforts and accomplishments during this period.

Near the close of the Middle Ages the church had lost much of its power, and monastic life no longer attracted young people. Therefore fewer persons were dedicated to the care of the sick. Several new orders were formed; one was the Beguines of Flanders, founded in 1184. This order devoted itself to the service of the sick and poor but functioned independently of church authority. As a result of the decreased number of practitioners, a great demand was created in the nursing field.

◆ The Decline of Nursing: Nursing from the Renaissance to the Nineteenth Century (1450-1800)

Although during the Renaissance Protestants urged the state to accept responsibility for the care of the sick, Catholics tried to salvage some of their nursing orders. At this time there were no experienced nurses to care for the ill except those within religious orders.

Because state officials showed little concern for hospitals established for the poor, hospitals and nursing care declined rapidly. It seems apparent that no sense of charity existed among the rich. When plague afflicted the people, the rich fled from the cities, leaving the poor without proper medication, food, and care. However, this period was not without magnanimous persons. John Howard (1727-1789), Mother Mary Catherine McAuley (1787-1841), and William Tuke (1732-1822) recognized the disastrous situation and attempted to reform nursing care and conditions in hospitals, prisons, and mental institutions. One of the outstanding men of this era, St. Vincent de Paul, dedicated his life as a priest to improving conditions for the sick. In 1600 he founded the Order of the Sisters of Charity with the assistance of Louise de Marillac. This order exists today, and its members continue to devote their time and efforts to the care of the poor and sick.

◆ The Beginning of Modern Nursing

Nursing Prior to Florence Nightingale

By the end of the eighteenth century nursing had reached its lowest ebb in Protestant countries. Educated women of the upper class disapproved of manual labor and no longer cared for the sick and needy. It was considered a disgrace to send a member of the family to the hospital; therefore the sick were cared for in the home.

Charles Dickens' novel *Martin Chuzzlewit* (1844), with its Sairey Gamp and Betsey Prig, best portrays nurses of this time as being women of immoral standards who were unsympathetic, alcohol-imbibing, and unfeeling individuals.

In Catholic communities in America the nursing situation was less devastating because priests and nuns who arrived with French and Spanish settlers possessed small amounts of nursing knowledge and skills. In Latin American countries nursing care was given by Catholic nursing orders. Hospitals existed in other countries long before they were established in the United States. The most commonly known orders in both North and South American hospitals were the Augustinian nuns, Ursuline nuns, and Sisters of Charity.

The first established school of nursing was founded in Kaiserswerth, Germany, in 1836 by a German pastor, Theodor Fliedner, who founded a hospital in his parish. With the assistance of an experienced nurse, Gertrude Reichardt, he revived the practice of deaconesses performing nursing functions. After 1 to 3 years of theory and practice the graduates of Kaiserswerth Deaconess Institution traveled to other parts of the world and founded similar programs. Florence Nightingale received her training at Kaiserswerth. Modern nursing begins with the Florence Nightingale era.

Nursing During the Florence Nightingale Era (1820-1910)

Florence Nightingale not only was the founder of modern nursing but also made it the respected career it is today. She was born of a wealthy family in Florence, Italy, on May 12, 1820. The year after her birth, Florence's family returned to England, and it was there she received her education. Despite her elite learning, social graces, and family opposition, Florence, possessed by a need to care for the sick, entered Kaiserswerth Deaconess Institution in 1851 to study nursing. She later worked and studied with the Sisters of Charity in Paris.

The first position held by Miss Nightingale was that of superintendent of a small institution in London, the Establishment for Gentlewomen During Illness. She worked diligently planning nursing care for her patients, and her efforts were rewarded. She was happy and successful. Florence strongly advocated that nursing existed for the healthy and for the sick.

When the Crimean War broke out, Russia and France had religious sisters to care for their wounded and sick, but England had only untrained men. Florence eagerly answered the call for help that came to her from the Secretary of War. On October 21, 1854, she set out with her small chosen group of nurses to serve her country and humanity.

In caring for the wounded soldiers Florence Nightingale met and tackled obstacles of filth, poor diet, understaffing, and inefficiency. She saw these deplorable conditions as a challenge and used her administrative genius in selecting nurses, erecting hospitals, and initiating much needed reforms. She provided the soldiers with clean bedding, nourishing food, hospital clothing, and skilled nurses to care for them. For her efforts she was honored with the title of Lady of the Lamp. Through her work during the war she broke down the age-old prejudice of the world toward nursing.

In 1862 William Rathbone begged Florence to assist him in establishing a home nursing service in London. Her response to this plea was the establishment of the

Training School and Home for Nurses of the Royal Infirmary. This program provided nurses for private duty, the hospital, and the district. This project marked the beginning of modern visiting nursing, better known today as *public health nursing*.

Florence Nightingale opened up the field of nursing as a profession. She was influential in establishing improved nursing programs and schools of nursing, improving woman's place in society and in the military, raising the standards of hospitals and facilities, and initiating the philosophy of "treating the patient rather than the disease." Florence served as the world's advisor on hospital matters and nursing service. She wrote many books; among her best known are *Notes on Nursing* and *Notes on Hospitals,* both published in 1859.

Florence Nightingale died in 1910 at age 90. Although she suffered criticisms and endured trials in order to succeed, her courage and stamina will be remembered forever. She saw nursing as a necessity and a challenge and fought for it. Her efforts were not in vain. Today nursing is the profession she wanted it to be.

Another outstanding nurse of the Florence Nightingale era was Ella King Newsom. Miss Newsom was Miss Nightingale's counterpart with the American Confederate Army. Ella Newsom received her training at Memphis City Hospital from the Sisters of Mercy and the medical staff. She applied her unusual organizational and executive abilities to erecting and administering hospitals while following the retreating Confederate Army. Her hospitals were noted for their cleanliness and humane treatment of the wounded.

◆ Nursing During the Late Nineteenth and Early Twentieth Centuries (1890-1960)

The greatest developments in modern nursing occurred during and after the Nightingale era, and nursing owes much to the leaders of this time. It was through their interest and tireless efforts that nursing advanced from an apprenticeship to a profession. It is difficult to read of the activities of these leaders without being caught up in the spirit that inspired and energized these dedicated persons.

Jean H. Dunant, a Swiss, formulated a plan of international relief for mass victims of war and calamity. The plan provided for independent associations and societies for war relief in each country with a strong international bond of affiliation among countries and a guaranteed neutrality of supplies and personnel. The plan was agreed on by representatives of 16 nations at the Geneva Conference in Switzerland in 1863. This agreement led to the formation of an International Red Cross Society. The society proposed to prepare in advance for war and disaster by gathering and storing all needed equipment such as medical and surgical supplies, clothing, portable shelters, furniture, and tools in large warehouses.

Because of the Civil War the United States was not present at the Geneva Conference and was the thirty-second country to enter the International Red Cross; thus the need to form a similar society in the United States, the American Red Cross Society, was recognized. This was accomplished through the tireless efforts of Clara Barton, a nurse in the Civil War. She organized the Red Cross Committee, based on Nightingale customs, in Washington and persuaded government officials to give the committee official standing in 1882. Clara Barton was the first president of the American Red Cross.

The Red Cross Society in the United States has given and loaned money and supplies to devastated areas and has helped rebuild houses or reestablish businesses. Outside the United States the organization has given supplies and aid in the reconstruction of countries where volcanic eruptions, floods, epidemics, and other disasters have occurred.

During this period medicine and nursing were making revolutionary strides. Louis Pasteur and Robert Koch introduced scientific discoveries and medical treatment based on bacteriological studies. Joseph Lister developed surgical antiseptic techniques that helped decrease the number of wound infections and deaths after surgical procedures. The process of nursing followed that of medicine, with a number of outstanding women giving greater dimension to the new profession.

Dorothea Dix, a retired schoolteacher, was a strong promoter of improving conditions and treatment of the mentally ill. Her first contact with the mentally ill was in a jail in East Cambridge, Massachusetts, in 1841. She was appalled at the environmental conditions existing in the jail where many mentally ill prisoners were held. Treatment of the prisoners ranged from indifference to brutality. She obtained data, secured the support of influential citizens, and presented these facts to government officials and to courts of law. Her efforts brought about improvements in jails and the establishment of psychiatric institutions.

To improve poor conditions existing in military camps, which included lack of care for sick soldiers and inadequacies of supplies, drugs, and transportation, Dorothea Dix was appointed Superintendent of the Female Nurses of the Army in 1861. Without military rank or a background of nurse's training, Miss Dix organized military hospitals, obtained needed materials, and supplied nurses to comfort and minister to the wounded and sick soldiers.

Linda Richards, the first trained nurse in America, graduated from the New England Hospital for Women and Children in Boston in 1872. After graduation her first assignment was night superintendent at Bellevue. One year later she was appointed superintendent of the Boston Training School. In addition to her teaching duties, she gave patient care and devoted long hours to the care of the sick. As a medical missionary in Japan from 1885 to 1889, Linda Richards established and directed the first training school for nurses in that country. Her remaining efforts were devoted to establishing nursing schools in hospitals for the mentally ill.

Near the turn of the century Isabel Hampton Robb (1860-1910) was linked with every type of organization, plan, and activity in nursing. She was a constructive thinker who could apply her ideas practically. In 1889 she initiated important reforms in nursing such as policies for a 12-hour day for student nurses; time allowance for meal, rest, study, and recreation periods; and a maximum limit to the workday. She helped eliminate private duty as part of the student nurse's education. In 1895 she advocated an 8-hour day for student nurses, the termination of stipends to raise the student nurse from the position of employee to that of student, and a 3-year nurse training program. She believed that licensing examinations and registration would protect patients from incompetent nurses and raise the status and standards of nurses. She was the first president of the Nurses Associated Alumnae of the United States and Canada, the first principal of the Johns Hopkins School of Nursing, and one of the founders and original stockholders of the *American Journal of Nursing*.

Mary Adelaide Nutting (1858-1947) was a graduate of the first class at the Johns Hopkins School of Nursing and a friend of Isabel Hampton Robb. She continued the reforms initiated by Mrs. Robb.

Her many accomplishments include separation of nursing schools from hospital ownership through state support for schools of nursing, raising the educational standards of basic nursing programs, founding nursing organizations, and creating and developing the Department of Nursing and Health at Teacher's College, Columbia University. She was honored with the title of First Professor of Nursing and was influential in the formation of the International Council of Nurses. In 1944 the National League of Nursing Education awarded Miss Nutting the first medal for leadership, the Adelaide Nutting Medal for Leadership in Nursing Education.

Lillian Wald (1867-1940) is best known as the foundress of the famed Henry Street Settlement. This event in 1893 marked the beginning of the development of the social service aspects of nursing as well as modern nursing in the community. The Henry Street Settlement, which began in a top-floor tenement on the Lower East Side of New York City, was established as a neighborhood nursing service for the sick poor. Lillian Wald's intensive crusade to assist the poor was based on her desire to nurse the poor as a friend rather than as a paid visitor. This was the true beginning of public health nursing in the United States.

Annie Goodrich (1876-1955) was the instigator of the Army School of Nursing in 1918. This school was founded as a war measure but designed to continue as a permanent organization. The 3-year course granted 9 months of credit to college graduates entering the program. The student's work was centered in army hospitals, and in 1920 officer's rank was granted to nurses.

In addition to Miss Goodrich's endeavors in the Army School of Nursing, she was president of the International Council of Nurses from 1912 to 1915, Director of the Visiting Nurse Service of the Henry Street Settlement in 1916, and Dean of Nursing at Yale.

Miss Nutting, Miss Wald, and Miss Goodrich are frequently referred to as The Great Trio in the rapid development of nursing during this period.

Mary E. Mahoney, America's first black graduate nurse, pressed for integration, better working conditions, and health care facilities in the Boston area. This pioneering nurse formed the National Association for Colored Graduate Nurses (NACGN).

Mildred L. Montag wrote her doctoral thesis, "Education of nursing technicians," proposing the establishment of a new position above the level of the practical nurse and below the level of the professional nurse. This position has been made possible by programs offered by the junior and community colleges. It is the Associate Degree of Nursing (ADN). These programs are scattered throughout the United States.

Another important person in nursing history is Isabel Maitland Stewart (1878-1963). Miss Stewart was influential in upgrading the educational status of nursing and in changing the thinking of nursing leaders both in the United States and abroad. She was the first nurse to receive a master's degree from Columbia University.

These dedicated nursing pioneers were totally involved in all aspects of nursing: military, international, educational, social, and public health. They were active in nursing organizations, reforms, and improvements. Their legacy to us can be found in their numerous writings.

Today nursing patterns are changing rapidly. Domestic tasks are no longer included in the duties of the registered nurse, who is assuming greater responsibility for the supervision of personnel, complicated medical and surgical procedures, and planning and implementing patient care in hospitals, homes, and community projects. The nurse is functioning in a leadership role. Nursing is now worldwide.

Space exploration has opened a new field for nurses; at the present this means caring for astronauts and their families, but in the future the nurse's role will expand to include numerous other facets in the aerospace program.

◆ Practical Nursing

The practical nurse became a permanent member of the health team when society needed a trained person who could render competent and intelligent bedside care to patients. The need for a training program for practical nurses was recognized early, and in 1893 the first school for practical nurses in the United States, the Ballard School, which consisted of a 3-month program, was founded in New York. Two other forerunners of the practical nursing schools of today were the Thompson School, founded in Brattleboro, Vermont, in 1907, and the Household Nursing Association School of Attendant Nursing, established in 1918 in Boston for the purpose of training practical nurses to give care in the home. Both of these schools are still in operation, although the Household Nursing Association School is now called the Shepard-Gill School of Practical Nursing. In our present system practical nursing programs are offered by hospitals, vocational-technical schools, and junior and community colleges.

In 1941, 28 people met in Chicago and formed the Association of Practical Nurse Schools. Hilda M. Torrop, Director of the Ballard School, Erta Creech, Director of the Family Health Association in Cleveland, and Katherine Shepard, Executive Director of the Household Nursing Association in Boston, were founders and officers of the association. Hilda Torrop later became the first executive director. In 1942 membership was opened to practical nurses, and the name of the association was changed to the National Association for Practical Nurse Education (NAPNE). In 1945 NAPNE established an accrediting service for practical nursing schools; it began holding a summer school and workshops for directors and instructors in 1950; and in 1951 it started the first practical nursing magazine, now called the *Journal of Practical Nursing*. By 1953 it was sponsoring summer continuing education programs for practical nurses. As time passed, the continuing education and welfare of practical nurses received more and more emphasis. In 1959 a Department of Service to State Practical Nursing Associations and a Department of Education were established, and the name of the association was changed to the National Association for Practical Nurse Education and Services (NAPNES).

In 1949 the National Federation of Licensed Practical Nurses (NFLPN) was organized by Lillian Kuster as the official membership organization for licensed practical nurses. Through the efforts of NAPNES and NFLPN the general public became aware of practical nursing, its educational programs, and the licensure of practical nurses.

In 1957 the Council on Practical Nursing (now Council of Practical Nursing Programs) was established under the auspices of the National League for Nursing (NLN) to help establish and maintain high-quality programs in schools of practical nursing, and in 1961 it became a department within the Division of Nursing Education. In 1962 the NFLPN founded the National Licensed Practical Nurses Educational Foundation for research, development of continuing education programs, and the awarding of scholarships to licensed practical nurses. It was through the combined efforts of NAPNES, NFLPN, and NLN that practical nursing became an integral part of nursing.

In 1979 the National League for Nursing councils developed, adopted, and published competencies of graduates of educational programs in practical nursing. Today practical nursing students are prepared by qualified nurse educators in structured health care settings such as hospitals. Clinical practice is correlated with basic therapeutic knowledge, mental health concepts, biological and behavioral sciences, and communication skills. Planned and supervised experiences are directed toward teaching students using current concepts and practices.

With the changes in the 1980s and 1990s, practical nurses are facing added responsibilities every day. The practical nurse now must assume more duties than ever before and make decisions during crises. We are in a time of rapid change that will continue.

In hospitals throughout the United States practical nurses make up a vital part of the organizational structure. Professional nurses are unable to function adequately without the assistance of practical nurses because of increased patient acuity, advances in technology, complexity of nursing care, and the demands of society. The function of the practical nurse is to render personalized bedside patient care and assist with care in complex situations. On successful completion of courses in an approved school, the practical nurse may function in the capacity of medicine nurse, team leader, or charge nurse.

Practical nurse programs do not prepare the nurse to go on to professional nursing, but in 1968 the NLN Council of Diploma Programs passed a resolution to make every effort to admit the LPN to diploma programs. This allows the LPN to challenge by examination those materials already learned and to move from one level of nursing to another with more ease. Since 1970 a greater effort has been made to allow LPNs to challenge course work through competency-based modules.

◆ *Study Helps*

1. Describe nursing as it existed in ancient civilizations.
2. Who was called the Father of Medicine, and why was he given this title?
3. How did the development of a middle class affect society and nursing in the Middle Ages?
4. Describe nursing during the Renaissance.
5. What contribution did St. Vincent de Paul make to the nursing profession?
6. Give a brief account of the life and activities of Florence Nightingale as they affected nursing.
7. What is the function of the Red Cross in the United States and abroad?
8. What were the chief contributions to nursing made by the following:
   - Dorothea Dix
   - Jean Dunant
   - Linda Richards
   - Clara Barton
   - Lillian Wald
   - Annie Goodrich
   - Mary Adelaide Nutting
   - Isabel Maitland Stewart
   - Isabel Hampton Robb
   - Hilda M. Torrop
   - Katherine Shepard
   - Etta Creech
   - Lillian Kuster
9. Which needs brought about the development of practical nursing?

Bibliography

Dolan JA: Nursing in society, ed 15, Philadelphia, 1982, WB Saunders Co.
Donahue MP: Nursing, the finest art, St Louis, 1985, The CV Mosby Co.
Fromer MJ: Ethical issues in health care, St Louis, 1981, The CV Mosby Co.
Marriner A: Nursing theorists and their work, St Louis, 1986, The CV Mosby Co.
Safier G: Contemporary American leaders in nursing: an oral history, New York, 1977, McGraw-Hill Book Co.
Saxton DF, Nugent PM, and Pelikan P: Mosby's comprehensive review of nursing, ed 12, St Louis, 1987, The CV Mosby Co.

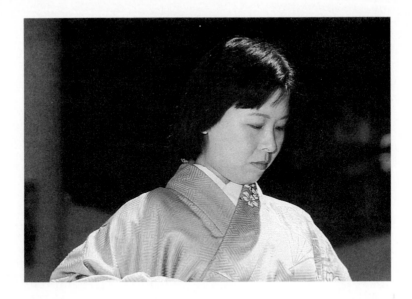

Objectives

At the completion of this chapter the student practical nurse will be able to:

◆ Identify the four ethnic-racial minorities.

◆ Summarize the spiritual needs of Catholics, Protestants, Jews, and other denominations.

4 Religions, Culture, and Ethnic Groups

Total patient care not only includes the physical care that you give to your patient during his illness but also spiritual care encompassing all religious groups. In some institutions there are routine visits by various religious representatives.

On routine visits or when a religious representative is called to visit a patient, you should extend every courtesy possible. Your assistance may be required; you must be understanding and helpful regardless of your own religious affiliations. You must respect your patient's wishes, ensure privacy, understand his religious practices, and prepare necessary articles for these practices to be carried out.

Some patients who have been indifferent to religion may find it very meaningful during illness. You are often the one who is asked to contact your patient's religious representatives; therefore one of your duties is to administer to your patient's spiritual needs.

The majority of Americans identify themselves as either Catholic, Protestant, or Jewish. Because of the variations in religions and the differences in patients' attitudes toward them, you must handle each one differently. You must know each patient's religious attitudes before you can offer intelligent and helpful assistance. A brief account of each of the major faiths may help you to understand better the various beliefs and attitudes of your patients.

Because of the unique practices and customs of Catholic and Jewish patients in the hospital setting, necessary details will be fully explained. These practices are founded on their beliefs. Therefore a knowledge and understanding of these beliefs must be obtained and understood to meet patients' spiritual needs adequately.

◆ Catholicism

Those of the Catholic faith recognize that their religion began with the birth of Jesus Christ. They believe that Christ is God, who lived as a human, suffered, and died for the spiritual welfare of the human race.

The Roman Catholic Church traces its foundation to Peter, one of the twelve apostles chosen by Jesus to carry on His work after His death. Peter, as the first official head of the church, passed down this line of authority to the present pontiff. The head of the Roman Catholic Church is known as the *pope*. There are also bishops and priests, whose principal functions are to preach and minister to the people of the church by means of seven sacraments. The seven sacraments of this church are baptism, confirmation, Holy Eucharist (Communion), reconciliation (confession), Holy Orders, matrimony, and sacrament of the sick. The four sacraments that you as a practical nurse will most commonly encounter in meeting the spiritual needs of your Catholic patients are baptism, reconciliation, Holy Eucharist, and sacrament of the sick.

Any time a Catholic patient is admitted to the hospital, the priest should be notified so that he may visit the patient. Regard the priest's visit as a means of fulfilling the spiritual needs of your patient, not as a sign of danger or impending death. When a priest is needed, you should call him as soon as possible, regardless of the time and without any delay. It is most desirable for the patient's and the family's peace of mind that the priest arrive while the patient is still conscious if at all possible.

Baptism

Because the Catholic patient believes that baptism is absolutely necessary for salvation, any adult, child, or newborn, including a miscarriage of a living fetus, must be baptized, if not previously baptized, when in danger of death. This emergency baptism may be performed by anyone if a priest is not available. It is preferable to have a Catholic physician or nurse, if present, baptize the patient. If this is not practical or possible, you may and should baptize the patient, regardless of your religion. The only prerequisite for administering this sacrament is that you have the desire to carry out the religious beliefs of this patient's religion; then you must perform the procedure correctly. The sacrament is administered by pouring water over the forehead of the patient or, if this is not possible, over any skin surface and saying *at the same time* these words: "I baptize you in the Name of the Father and of the Son and of the Holy Spirit."

If you have any doubt as to whether the patient is still alive or has been baptized before, administer the sacrament conditionally. This is done by prefixing the baptismal words: "If you are capable of being baptized, I baptize you in the Name of the Father. . . ." By using the word *capable*, you include the facts that the patient is still alive, that he has the right disposition to receive the sacrament if he is an adult, and that he has never been baptized before. It is important to remember that the words must be said at the *same* time as you are pouring the water. The water must touch the skin itself, meaning that if there is any secretion, drainage, or foreign material on the skin, it must be cleansed before pouring the water. The hospital chaplain should be notified later that the emergency baptism was administered to the patient.

Mass

To assist at Mass on Sundays and holy days of obligation is the first commandment of the Catholic Church. Catholics pay homage to God by their participation in the liturgy of the Mass, which is the central prayer of the Catholic religion. A person may have a legitimate excuse such as illness or an emergency for not attending Mass on Sundays or holy days.

In the hospital setting your patient may want to attend Mass in the hospital chapel if the hospital has one. If the patient's condition warrants attendance and permission of the attending physician has been obtained, assist your patient to the chapel either in a wheelchair or by walking, depending on his physical condition.

If unable to attend Mass, some patients like to read prayer books or recite prayers in the hospital room to fulfill this obligation. Some may desire to watch a televised Mass on Sunday mornings. In these cases you should give them adequate privacy.

It is a good point to remember that hospitalized patients are not obligated to attend Sunday Mass. The fact that they have been admitted to the hospital excuses them from this obligation. However, the patient's conscience, his physical condition, and the necessary medical permission should be the guiding factors in making this decision. A Catholic patient should never be forced to attend Sunday Mass or be judged for not attending this service.

Reconciliation

The sacrament of reconciliation is also referred to as *confession* or *penance*. In this sacrament Catholics seek reconciliation with God by expressing sorrow for their offenses against God or others. The priest offers a sign of this forgiveness through the words of absolution. It is advisable to ask a Catholic patient if he would like to see a priest on admission to the hospital, before going to surgery, in case of an accident, or in any critical illness. Privacy should be ensured, and the priest should be provided with a chair so that he may talk with the patient. To a Catholic patient this sacrament may be a form of therapy as valuable as medication and treatment.

Holy Eucharist

Holy Eucharist, or Communion, is regarded as another important sacrament for the Catholic patient because he believes that he receives by way of bread and wine, the Body and Blood, Soul and Divinity of Jesus Christ. Communion is usually received frequently but *must* be received during the Easter season. Communion is always given, if possible, when there is danger of death and may be requested by the patient before going to the operating room.

A priest should be called any time a Catholic patient is in danger of death, regardless of whether or not he is a practicing Catholic. If the patient is capable of receiving Holy Communion, he may do so at this time.

Sacrament of the Sick

The sacrament of the sick consists of anointment with holy oils. It is given to all those who have a serious illness or are facing serious surgery. Usually the priest and patient together make the decision; however, a priest should be called at the family's request or if the nurse sees a marked deterioration in the patient's condition. If a patient is unconscious, a priest should be called and given the details of the individual's condition.

Food Practices

The rules of fasting and abstinence have been changed; fasting is now voluntary. Ash Wednesday and Good Friday are the only days requiring complete fasting and abstinence. However, you will discover some patients who prefer to follow the older practices. According to the older practice, fasting restricts persons between the ages of 21 and 60 to one full meal a day with limitations placed on the other meals. Abstinence restricts the use of meat for those 14 years of age or older every Friday, on ember days, and on other designated vigils.

◆ Protestantism

Episcopalians, Methodists, Lutherans, Presbyterians, Baptists, members of the United Church of Christ, and Seventh-Day Adventists are classified as Protestants. Although these denominations have differences, they have many beliefs in common. These differences and beliefs will be briefly noted.

Episcopalians

Episcopalians profess many of the Catholic beliefs but do not recognize the pope as Christ's vicar and head of the church. Private confession exists but is not compulsory. Episcopalians follow the Bible as a guide but do not hold to exact interpretation. They believe in heaven and hell but do not believe that heaven and hell exist as places. They make and observe laws concerning divorce and birth control. They use Holy Unction for those in danger of death but more often as a sacrament of healing. Episcopalian patients often like to receive Holy Communion. They believe baptism should be performed if an infant shows signs of dying.

Methodists

Methodists believe that religion is a personal matter. They believe that it is what a person feels. Conscience dictates their actions. They force changes when they believe changes are needed. The Methodist religion will accept baptism of all other denominations. They accept baptism by sprinkling or by immersion into water in either infancy or adulthood. They do not believe in canonization of saints or in purgatory. They believe that after death the good will be rewarded and the evil will be punished. They have flexible laws concerning divorce and birth control.

Lutherans

The Lutheran religion accepts the Trinity and regards Christ as both God and man. They believe that faith is the integral part of religion. Confirmation is considered a rite, not a sacrament, in their religion. Their practiced sacraments are baptism (by sprinkling for both children and adults) and Communion. They believe that the presence of Christ is real in Communion.

Presbyterians

Presbyterians emphasize sovereignty of one God in three persons. They believe in the Bible and in heaven and hell. They believe that salvation cannot be obtained by living a good life because it is a gratuitous gift from God. They practice the sacraments of baptism (usually sprinkling) and Communion. They believe that Christ is present in spirit in Communion.

Baptists

Baptists, historically, are not Protestants because they existed as a denomination before the Reformation by Martin Luther. However, they are often classified as Protestants. The Baptists have no formal creed but emphasize that Christ heads the church. They restrict baptism to those old enough to understand its meaning. They practice total immersion. They take Communion as a remembrance of Christ's death. They often confess their sins openly before the congregation and ask forgiveness in this way. However, this method is not mandatory.

United Church of Christ

The United Church of Christ, the result of a union in 1957 of the Evangelical and Reformed Church and the Congregational Christian Church, bases its beliefs and teachings on Holy Scripture. Practices include infant baptism, with full communicant church membership beginning at ages 12 to 14. The sacrament of the Lord's Supper is open to all Christian believers. Its policy is understanding of, respect for, and cooperation with all Christian groups.

Seventh-Day Adventists

The Seventh-Day Adventist religion is basically Protestant. Their members are usually vegetarians. They do not believe in infant baptism. This denomination believes in study and devotional readings of the Bible, both individually and in groups. They believe in public and private worship, emphasizing prayer. They require their members to carry out the teachings of the Bible, as interpreted by the leaders of the churches and by the individual person.

Background and Baptism

Baptism, as essential for salvation, is not the belief of some Protestant denominations. They believe in the right of the individual to choose the type of religion he believes meets his own needs in dealing with God. Certain institutions may be referred to as "ordinances in another religion."

A Protestant minister should be contacted anytime, day or night, if his presence is requested by the patient or by the patient's family. It is best if the clergyman arrives while the patient is still conscious or before he has received any sedation.

When a patient believes that baptism is essential to salvation and there is any doubt as to whether the minister will arrive in time, then you as a practical nurse may baptize an adult or child who has not been baptized. There must be a witness or sponsor present who should be another baptized person if possible. While baptizing the patient, the practical nurse must make sure the water touches the skin, while saying the words: "(The patient's name if known), I baptize you in the Name of the Father and of the Son and of the Holy Spirit." The words must be said while the water is being poured on the forehead or, if this is impossible, any other part of the body.

Emergency baptism should be reported to the proper person so that the family can be notified that it was performed (if this is feasible). Baptism should be recorded on the patient's chart, in the nurse's notes, or on the admission sheet or Kardex, as indicated by the policy of the respective hospital.

◆ Other Christian Denominations

There are other Christian denominations that are not Catholic or Protestant. Some of these are Jehovah's Witnesses, Friends (Quakers), Christian Scientists, the Eastern Orthodox Church, and the Church of Jesus Christ of Latter-Day Saints. These denominations will be briefly presented.

Jehovah's Witnesses

Jehovah's Witnesses stress one God (Jehovah). Their beliefs come from the Bible. The beliefs of these people prevent them from receiving whole blood, blood plasma, or any blood derivative.

Friends (Quakers)

The Society of Friends (Quakers) has no ministers. Spiritual needs are met through members of the meeting. They have individual interpretations and practices.

Christian Scientists

Christian Scientists believe in spiritual healing. These patients are usually taken care of in one of their church-operated nursing homes or at home. If a Christian Scientist is admitted to a hospital because of an emergency, a Christian Science practitioner should be contacted. If a Christian Scientist is admitted to the hospital through a private physician, the written orders of the physician are to be followed.

Eastern Orthodox Church

Because the Eastern Orthodox Church has many of the same beliefs and practices as the Roman Catholic Church, it is wise to check to see which religious representative should be notified.

The Church of Jesus Christ of Latter-Day Saints (Mormonism)

This religion was organized by Joseph Smith in 1830. The Mormons believe in the Bible, as translated by the Mormon Church, the Book of Mormon, as the word of God, the gifts of prophecy, healing, and revelation, and return of Christ to rule the earth in person. They practice the rites of baptism and the Lord's Supper. They maintain an extensive welfare program to assist needy members and support numerous missionaries overseas. In some cases of emergency the welfare recipients need not make repayment. Members of this religion do not believe in infant baptism. Their health laws do not allow tea, coffee, cola, alcohol, or tobacco. They do not believe in deathbed repentance but do believe in anointing the patient with olive oil before performing procedures and in asking a blessing for the patient.

◆ Judaism

The Jewish religious year is based on a lunar calendar instead of the solar calendar. The Jewish faith is based on the five books of Moses, called the *Torah*. The Jewish religion follows the teachings of Moses. Today there are three types of Jewish groups. The Orthodox group is the oldest and the most resistant to ritualistic change. The Conservative group is less resistant to ritualistic change. The Reform group is the modern group that often makes deliberate changes in its ritual. The Jewish representative is known as the *rabbi*. He is the one to be contacted for a Jewish patient.

The Sabbath

The Sabbath, observed from sunset Friday until after sunset Saturday, is a day for prayer, rest, and study. Services are held on Friday evenings and Saturday mornings. The Sabbath meal is an important observance. The family may have a lighting-of-candles ritual. This may be requested by some patients.

Food Practices

Food practices vary according to whether the patient is Orthodox, Conservative, or Reformed. The "kosher" practice is observed by the Orthodox group, the Conservative group, and some Reformed Jews. In the kosher practice the main dietary laws involve utensils, meats, fish, and dairy products.

The utensils are kept in two separate groups; one group is used to prepare meat dishes and the other to prepare dishes containing dairy products. These utensils include dishes, silverware, and pans. When a set of glassware is used, it must be cleansed in a special way between uses.

Meat must come from divided-hoofed mammals such as cows, antelope, goats, and deer. These mammals must chew a cud. Other meats that may be eaten can come from any fowl, such as turkeys, geese, and chickens, but must exclude any birds of prey. All meats must be slaughtered and prepared in a kosher way; all blood must be removed.

Fish that have both scales and fins do not come under the regulation of meat. They may be eaten with either dairy products or meat if they are prepared with a vegetable shortening.

Dairy products are not eaten with or after a meat meal. Eggs are an exception and may be served with meat. Vegetables may be used as a substitute for meat.

Today many food products are manufactured in accordance with kosher dietary standards and these foods are marked with a ⓤ. Foods marked as *pareve* (neither meat nor dairy product) may be served with meat or dairy products.

The *Kosher Products Directory* is published annually and may be obtained free from the Union of Orthodox Jewish Congregations of America.

When the physician believes that fasting would endanger the patient's life, the patient will be excused from observing a fast.

Circumcision

Circumcision is a religious custom that takes place on the eighth day after birth unless contraindicated for medical reasons. This is a religious custom with prescribed rituals. At this time the boy receives his name. An obstetrician or surgeon may perform the circumcision on a Reformed Jew, with the rabbi reading certain prayers. Female children are named in their parents' house of worship, with the rabbi saying appropriate prayers.

Bar Mitzvah (boys), Bas Mitzvah (girls)

Bar mitzvah and bas mitzvah are ceremonies celebrated after a boy's and girl's thirteenth birthday. These ceremonies signify religious maturity.

Jewish Holidays

Some of the Jewish holidays are Rosh Hashanah, Yom Kippur, Succoth, Hanukkah, Passover, and Shavuoth. These holidays will be briefly explained.

Rosh Hashanah. Rosh Hashanah is a High Holiday; it is also the Jewish New Year. This is a day in autumn when God judges the deeds of man.

Yom Kippur. Yom Kippur is the Day of Atonement and is celebrated 10 days after the Jewish New Year. This holiday is celebrated by fasting and prayer and ends the penitence period.

Succoth. Succoth is similar to the solar calendar day of Thanksgiving. This holiday is celebrated for 9 days and ends with selected readings from Jewish scripture.

Hanukkah. Hanukkah falls near the solar calendar day of Christmas and is celebrated for 8 days with the lighting of candles.

Passover. Passover falls near the solar calendar of Easter. This holiday is celebrated for 8 days with special foods (unleavened breads) and services.

Shavuoth. Shavuoth is celebrated in commemoration of receiving the Ten Commandments and may be confirmation day for Jewish adolescents.

Death Procedures

Death procedures will vary according to the three Jewish groups. The Orthodox and Conservative Jews do not believe in autopsies. They believe that a person near death should not be left alone. Even in the Reform group, usually members of the family and the rabbi will stay with a dying person. The Orthodox and Conservative groups do not believe in embalming. Therefore, if possible, the funeral is held before sundown on the day the patient dies. They do not believe in burial on the Sabbath and certain holidays. They believe in sitting Shiva for 7 days after a death.

All these rules have been altered in the Reformed group to spare the feelings of the saddened family and to give support and consolation.

If no specific instructions as to the burial ceremonies have been received, then the body should be prepared according to hospital procedure.

◇   ◇   ◇

Religion plays an important part in the lives of most people; therefore, the spiritual leaders join the team of the hospital staff in meeting the patient's needs. As a practical nurse you should be familiar with the various religions so that you can carry through your important role in meeting the complete needs of your patients.

Table 2 ◇ *Summary of religious rites and practices*

Jewish	Protestant	Roman Catholic
Death and autopsy		
Family or rabbi will make arrangements for burial Because some Jews object to autopsy, consult rabbi or family regarding autopsy	Most Protestant denominations administer last sacraments, if they believe in them, before death occurs No moral objection to autopsy	Roman Catholics should receive, if possible and desirable, sacrament of the sick, penance, and Holy Eucharist Ritual should be performed during illness or before death No moral objection to autopsy
Conditions involving serious illnesses		
May not desire surgical procedure performed on Sabbath or holy day May desire to see rabbi	May desire to see minister to pray and talk Minister will determine whether patient is to receive Holy Communion, confession, or Extreme Unction	When ill or in danger of death, patient may desire to receive penance, Holy Communion, and sacrament of the sick Chaplain or parish priest will administer sacraments as determined by condition and desire of patient

◆ Culture

Culture is the customary beliefs, material traits, and social forms of a religious, racial, or social group. Recognition of cultural differences is very important in understanding the behavior of ourselves and others. Culture refers to human activities that are passed from one generation to the next. It applies to the collective ways of life in a group of people. It includes some basics such as language, diet, family support groups, religion, mating, government, wars, clothing, shelter, and daily life. No two cultures are exactly alike, although most have similar fundamental needs. The cultural characteristics of a group may or may not be exhibited by every individual in that group.

Subcultures are fairly large numbers of people, who, although members of a larger cultural group, have shared characteristics that are not common to all members of the culture. For example, because of their knowledge and skills, practical nurses belong to a subculture.

◆ Ethnic Groups

Ethnicity refers to races or large groups of people classed according to common traits and customs. In the United States, ethnic groups are based on the following factors: religion, race, language, politics, and nationality. These factors differentiate minority groups in our society.

Because you are human, you may be affected by the prejudices of others. You may even have some prejudices of your own. Acceptance of the fact that all persons are created equal, regardless of their race, may help you to overcome prejudices and better meet your patients' needs.

Race has become difficult to classify because of populations' mobility, intermarriage, and intermixing of cultures, which blend races so that no line can be drawn between any two of them. Humans have been divided into the following three major races by some anthropologists:

1. Mongolian race, which is made up of most of the people of the Far East, such as the Japanese and Chinese
2. Negro or black race, which is made up of most dark-skinned people, such as those of African descent
3. Caucasian or white race, which is made up of light-skinned people who share certain physical features, such as most people from Europe, the Middle East, and part of the East Indies

You may hear groups called the "Jewish race" or the "American race," but these are incorrect. These groups are not races but a religious group and a national group, respectively.

The distinguishing characteristics of races are minor physical differences such as skin color, facial features, and body size. The changes have probably come about through a natural process of evolution, in which individuals have changed to adjust to their environmental conditions. Physical differences are the only ones that can be found. The main racial stocks have been mixing so that no definite line can be drawn between any two races. No race is better or more intelligent than another. Given equal social, educational, economic, and environmental backgrounds, each race will parallel the achievements of the other races.

Proof of this statement can be found in the life of Mary Eliza Mahoney, the first black nursing graduate. From a class of forty, only three students graduated in 1879 from the 16-month course given at the New England Hospital for Women and Children. Miss Mahoney was one of the three graduates and the only black student in her class. Her fine record at school, skill, devotion, and intelligence in pursuing her nursing vocation in Boston after graduation furthered intergroup relationships and paved the way for blacks to achieve a place in nursing.

In 1909 she gave the welcoming address at the first conference of the National Association of Colored Graduate Nurses. In 1936 this Association initiated the Mary Mahoney Medal in her honor. The medal serves as a symbol of the opportunities in nursing for individuals of all races, creeds, and nationalities.

As a nurse you are responsible for your patient's well-being, regardless of his race, nationality, or religion. Every person has rights. You should never be convinced by anyone that this is not true. You must safeguard the patient's rights, regardless of your feelings or those of others, for all humans are equal.

◆ *Study Helps*

1. Why is it necessary to know and understand the religious beliefs of your patients?
2. What are the beliefs of the Catholic religion?
3. How would you meet the spiritual needs of a critically ill or dying Catholic patient?
4. How is conditional baptism administered?
5. Why is the Holy Eucharist so important to the Catholic patient?
6. What are the current regulations with regard to fasting and abstinence for the modern-day Catholic?
7. Which denominations are classified under Protestantism? Briefly describe each denomination's beliefs and practices.
8. What is the basis of the Jewish religion? What are its religious practices and customs?
9. Who was the first black nurse?
10. What does the Mary Mahoney Medal symbolize?
11. Define *culture*.

Bibliography

Collins M: Communications in health care, ed 2, St Louis, 1983, The CV Mosby Co.

Cox ML: 1981, Notes from the chairperson, Council on Intercultural Nursing Newsletter, 1:1.

Orque MS, Bloch B, and Monrroy LSA: Ethnic nursing care, St Louis, 1983, The CV Mosby Co.

Primeaux M and Henderson G: Transcultural health care, Reading, Mass, 1981, Addison-Wesley Publishing Co.

Saxton DF, Nugent PM, and Pelikan P: Mosby's comprehensive review of nursing, ed 12, St Louis, 1987, The CV Mosby Co.

Smith H: The religions of man, New York, 1961, Mentor Books.

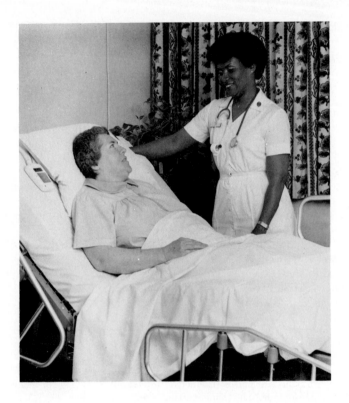

Objectives

At the completion of this chapter the student practical nurse
will be able to:

◆ Define self-awareness.

◆ List ways in which the nurse can assist the patient to adjust
  to a strange environment.

◆ Differentiate responsibilities of the registered nurse from those
  of the practical nurse.

◆ List five patient rights.

Role of the Practical Nurse

♦ **Getting Acquainted with a New Way of Life and a Rapidly Changing Vocation**

When someone speaks of a "new way of life," what immediately comes to your mind? Do you think of something different, challenging, starting over? Some people accept change as long as it does not disturb the humdrum routines of their daily lives. Almost everyone knows that change is inevitable if one is to grow in depth and scope. Some people want change to come about without too much effort on their part. Others are thrilled by the challenge that a change may present. Change, with its varying experiences, is similar to an adventure in the unknown. Such an adventure takes its toll on your entire being; it affects you physically, psychologically, emotionally and perhaps even spiritually. If the outcome of an adventure is good and what you had hoped for, you are pleased. On the other hand, if the adventure proves to be a failure, you are disappointed.

You may regard practical nursing as a "new way of life" or a "new beginning." Practical nursing is an integral part of nursing, a scientific and personal service rendered to community members with specific health needs. It requires sacrifice, willingness, and selflessness. To give of yourself in this capacity, you need to know yourself, and that is probably one of the most difficult things in life. It requires looking into yourself, knowing who, what, where, and why you are on this earth. It is a self-awareness, and it can help you to recognize your strengths and your limitations. Self-awareness helps you to get in touch with your philosophy for living and your set of values. These will be basic to your functioning as a person and as a nurse. Knowing yourself will also make you more self-confident and more comfortable with your self-image. A study of yourself is not an overnight process; you cannot change immediately, although you may like to. Traits are developed from childhood and throughout life. You did not grow from infancy to adulthood in 24 hours or even a week; therefore you cannot expect or demand immediate change within yourself. A continual striving on your part will cause these changes to occur gradually.

As you enter nursing, your new way of life, how can you become acquainted with it? Nursing is not something abstract. It is something real—a service performed to and for real people. The people who are the closest to you as you enter training are your fellow student nurses and your instructors. You come into contact with them before you reach the patient. You learn from them, with them, and through them. Your goal is to become an efficient practical nurse capable of rendering quality patient care. This implies that you give your best and that you know yourself well. But how can you do this? At first you must rely on your imagination, past learning, judgment, and memory. Later your companions and instructors can help you. Frequently it is others who help you most if only you will allow yourself to learn from and through them. It can be your opportunity to grow to your fullest and become a mature individual. Maturity is expected in professionals. Therefore you must strive to know your companions and instructors, and, in turn, you will become better acquainted with yourself. These relationships can assist you to better understand the needs of your patients and enable you to administer quality patient care.

Thus far it has been mentioned that you must know yourself better and work through your fellow student nurses and instructors to bring about this effect. Other factors and persons involved in becoming acquainted with this new way of life include the patient, the patient's relatives, and the hospital itself. All these factors greatly influence your behavior and adjustment.

First, consider the patient. What is his reaction to you? What is his role in the hospital? The patient is an ill person who has been transported from his own environment to an entirely new environment to which he must adjust. The patient identifies the hospital and each member of the health team as one. Ordinarily he does not make a distinction between the graduate nurse, the practical nurse, the nursing assistant, the x-ray technician, or any other member of the health team. He regards you as one who is directly responsible for his immediate care and recovery. He watches your every movement, your responses to his illness and the symptoms he manifests, and your actions and dealings with other patients. He judges you in view of these manifestations to assure himself that he is in capable hands and will recover through your efficient, kind, and conscientious care.

The patient is also fearful. The hospital setting may be foreign to him. The patient does not know what is expected of him in the hospital's routine. You can allay some of these fears if you take time to explain things the patient needs to know. For example, you may tell him to go down the hall to take a shower. "Down the hall" to the patient may mean going to another nursing division, which may be a distance down the hall, or it may mean several doors from his room. It is simpler to say to him, "Mr. Jones, the bathroom or shower is five doors down the corridor on the right-hand side." This short explanation clearly describes the location of the bathroom and allays the patient's anxiety and fear of the unknown. It is easy for you to take things for granted, especially after you have become accustomed to the hospital setting. It becomes a second home to you, but when you started as a new student, you were often frustrated. Your instructors helped you to overcome this frustration, but who is to help the patient?

As a student practical nurse you will spend much time at the bedside. You will have the opportunity to become acquainted with the patient and to explain details to him that are often taken for granted and assumed that he knows. Be empathetic to the patient. Empathy is an attempt to experience the individual's emotional state as if you were in the individual's place. It allows the patient's world to become the nurse's world for a time. Such involvement helps nurses to see patients as they are and not as they "ought" to be. It helps the nurse to become more appreciative of the feelings of others.

The nurse must establish a personalized type of communication with the patient. This can be difficult with someone you do not know or if there is a difference in age, sex, race, or culture. People usually interpret what is communicated according to their customary ways of thinking and their patterns of experience. The nurse, in these matters, must remain objective to prevent personal values from changing the meaning of the message. The patient has been taken from the home situation and placed in the hospital setting. The patient knows exactly where everything is at home, but in the hospital things are in different places. There are favorite television programs that are watched routinely, but the patient may not even have a television in his room. The patient may be in a double room with a person who appears very ill and who may die. Immediately the concern and thinking begins, "I wonder if they'll find that I have something serious and that I'll die too." The other patient may not be acutely ill but merely appears so to the new patient. The two may remain strangers to each other because no one has introduced them. When you entered training, you may have had to introduce yourself to your companions, and this may have been very difficult for you. Perhaps you even shied away from others, and then you were very lonely. A patient frequently experiences these same problems when he is admitted to a hospital, but they can be minimized if hospital personnel are friendly and nurses take the time to explain things to the patient.

The patient also feels that at home his friends can visit as often and as long as they desire. In the hospital restrictions are placed on visitors. They are told exactly when they may visit. Occasionally they are not treated in as friendly a manner as they should be treated. Examples of unfriendly treatment of visitors follow:

1. You enter the room to perform some particular patient procedure and find that the patient has visitors. Because you are hurried as a result of having much to do, you appear curt and say as few words as possible, such as "Please leave the room."

2. On entering the room and finding the patient has visitors, you turn around and walk out without saying a word.

Neither the patient nor his visitors would object if you were to ask the visitors in a pleasant voice to wait in the hall or in the waiting room for a few minutes. You could simply explain that you wish to perform some procedure for the patient. It would be much better to say, "Hello, Mr. Jones, I see that you have visitors. I have a procedure to do that can wait; I'll return when visiting hours are over." This approach allows the patient and his visitors to feel comfortable with you. They feel accepted by you and are more willing to cooperate with you. A few words and gestures can make a great deal of difference. If you were in a fellow student's room and another student walked in suddenly, saw you, and left immediately without saying anything, you would feel uncomfortable. The patient experiences these same feelings.

The patient is a very knowledgeable consumer. He is aware of the cost of a hospital and will expect services equal to that cost. Hospital and personnel will often be judged by the quality of care rendered. Therefore it is important that the patient is made to feel secure and safe and to know that he will be cared for in a concerned and empathetic manner. Hospital personnel are "ambassadors of good will." Their behavior and the care they administer will often enhance or negate the reputation of a health facility.

As a practical nurse you would not want to work in any hospital that does not have a good reputation for service. It is important to remember, however, that no matter how beautiful a structure is, the spirit in which a nurse administers patient care is what really counts.

When you are not feeling well, what is the first thing you attack or criticize? It is frequently the food. The ill patient reacts similarly. Every effort should be made by dietary personnel to ensure the patient is served a tray of appetizing food. Because his activities are limited, the patient has little to do but wait from meal to meal. If the meal arrives and he receives food he did not order or silverware is missing from the tray, he is greatly disappointed. If his tray does not arrive at all, the patient becomes angry. Perhaps no one thought to tell the patient that his tray was being held or omitted because of some type of test. If he had been informed, he would have accepted this calmly and patiently.

The patient's feelings and reactions to you and your reactions to the patient will be discussed in more detail in later chapters.

For the present you should acquaint yourself with the hospital. The hospital may be a large or small institution. Regardless of size it is simply a structure filled with many skilled people, ranging from the administrator of the hospital to the janitor, the housekeeping department, and the laundry. It consists of various departments, each with a specific purpose. Each department affects the patient and you, either directly or indirectly. If one department fails to do an efficient job, then everyone feels the effects of this failure. The hospital contains large quantities of different types of equipment. Each has its specific function and it may benefit you to learn as much as you can about it. For example, if the electrocardiogram machine is not operated correctly or handled carefully by the technician, it will lose its sensitivity. As a result of this sensitivity loss, the patient's heart waves will be recorded inaccurately. This may prove costly to the patient in terms of an incorrect diagnosis and to the hospital as a financial loss.

You will learn the various departments and their functions through lectures, classes, and your working relationships. You can become acquainted with the hospital personnel through a friendly hello when you meet them in the cafeteria, in their respective departments, or in the corridors. Remember, as a member of the nursing team, you belong to the entire hospital team; you should know these persons and their functions.

◆ Practical Nursing

Practical nursing plays an important part in the total nursing program, and the practical nurse has a definite role to play. This role is to give quality nursing care to patients or groups of patients at home or in institutions, under the supervision of a registered nurse or licensed physician. The advances made in research and therapy and the rapid strides made in nursing have caused the duties of the practical nurse to change. In the future, responsibility for performing more detailed and specialized types of nursing care will be given to the practical nurse. To prepare the student practical nurse for this role, practical nursing programs have revised curricula to make them more comprehensive and have employed better-prepared faculties. Today's practical nurse can find career opportunities in numerous fields such as public health, industry, the military, and home health agencies; these fields are discovering the need for and worth of practical nurses and are welcoming them.

Knowledge is basic to all professions. Because practical nursing is comprehensive, you are required to take many courses in theory and practice to provide you with the knowledge and information essential to your vocation. This means that you must study and learn to the best of your ability all the subject matter that is essential to the program. You have the legal obligation to become a well-informed practitioner of nursing because your lack of knowledge may someday be detrimental to the safety of patient. Beyond the legal obligation, your desire to care for the sick and infirm spurs you on to acquire the knowledge and skill of practical nursing. This desire may be an integral part of your character; it may have come from your association with other practical nurses who have been your friends or someone who deeply impressed you when a member of your family required hospitalization. The end result is that you want and are now studying to become a practical nurse.

As you become more familiar with nursing, you will discover that it is not the glamorous life that some may think. It is hard work, but it is rewarding. You can find your greatest satisfaction in rendering quality nursing care to those in need. You must find fulfillment in your work; otherwise you will not work to your fullest capacity.

◆ The Practical Nurse Today

What does the word *nurse* mean? A nurse is an educationally prepared and technically skilled person capable of rendering competent scientific and personal care to the sick and to those in need. The registered nurse assumes responsibility for the nursing care given to patients and develops an effective collaboration with various other health practitioners. At one time the registered nurse was function oriented; it is now concerned with a more demonstrative role in assisting patients to meet their psychosocial needs. Emphasis is now placed on the total care of the patient, on compassion and understanding, and on accepting the patient as he is. The practical nurse works under the supervision of the registered nurse and renders direct nursing care in less complex situations and assists with the nursing care in more complex situations. Less complex situations are those of a more stable and nonacute nature. In these situations, the practical nurse can function independently and provide much of the actual bedside care. Complex situations refer to those circumstances requiring specialized knowledge and judgment in caring for critically ill patients. In these situations, the practical nurse who has close contact with the patient assesses his basic needs, alleviates his physical discomforts, and reports any abnormal findings to the registered nurse or attending physician.

In this book the terms *practical nurse* and *vocational nurse* are used interchangeably. In some states the former type of nurse is called a vocational nurse; in others the title is practical nurse.

In the capacity of a practical nurse you fulfill not only the patient's needs but also your own. When you administer bedside patient care, provide comfort to the patient, and note results such as the alleviation of pain, you feel satisfied with yourself and rewarded for your efforts. You also have the satisfaction of forming a close relationship with the patient that is warm and comforting. You learn empathy, which means that you are able to feel as the patient feels without actually going through the ordeal of disease and suffering that the patient is experiencing.

If you want to become a good nurse, which qualifications and abilities should you possess? You should be dependable and trustworthy. Think back to the people with whom you have come in contact or whom you know. Which trait is admired most and greatly missed if absent? Many would choose the trait of dependability. Everyone wants to be able to rely on someone. If a friend says something is to be done, you know that it will be done. You, as a practical nurse, need to develop a high degree of dependability. The patient, members of the nursing team, and the physician expect this of you. You must be able to assess the situation and know how, when, and where to perform a procedure or treatment safely, carefully, and thoroughly. A trait that goes hand in hand with dependability is trust. Trust is a firm belief or confidence in the integrity, reliability, honesty, and justice of another person. The patient and the family trust you to do your best to assist in the recovery process, if possible. You need to have perseverance and determination to do a job well. Regardless of how difficult the job may become or how many obstacles you must overcome, you should have the stamina and ability to accomplish it. You may not like the job, but you should complete it to the best of your ability.

The nurses who are admired most are cheerful and caring. They have a reverence for life and an appreciation of humanity. They establish a rapport with the patient and listen carefully to what the patient has to say. They share a part of the patient's life and participate in his joy when an illness is prevented or when a recovery occurs. The caring nurse shares a part of a family's grief when death occurs or some of the happiness when a young child is told he will need no more injections. The practical nurse cannot solve all the problems of the patient but by listening can frequently help the patient think through problems calmly, logically, and thoroughly. The cheerful nurse who is willing to listen brings happiness to the patient. Who does not want a bit of sunshine when everything is overcast and cloudy?

Nursing personnel are expected to be kind, and patients are disappointed when they are not. Patients often forget that nurses are human and that everyone fails at times or has personal problems. The people who are remembered the longest are those who were the kindest. A gentle pat on the shoulder when feeling down, a kind word when feeling hurt, or a warm handshake when feeling rejected by friends or family may be all that is needed. Because your work as a nurse is directed to the care of the sick, kindness is a must in your life. Normal feelings become exaggerated in the patient who is suffering from illness. Kindness can be the buffer for these feelings.

In every institution, whether it is a school, hospital, or business, someone is given governing authority. This authority gives a person the right to direct, guide, and make decisions. In the nursing situation you are expected to follow the orders of the registered nurse and physician. The fact that you consent to work in an institution means that you are willing to follow the rules and regulations of that particular institution. This means that you do not alter, change, or neglect a procedure that you do not like. It means that you are conscientious in observing proper procedure.

Rules are made to ensure order and uniformity, to safeguard the institution, and to ensure the best care for the patient. For example, a physician knows that early ambulation is necessary to ensure full range of motion and healing. If the nurse decides that this order is severe and ambulates the patient only once a day, this decision can have serious consequences for the patient. It may necessitate a repeat operation, a prolonged hospital stay, or failure of complete recovery without full range of motion. The patient needs to be assured that all personnel are working for his improvement and that orders written by his physician will be carried out accurately. The physician, who has the full responsibility for the medical care of the patient, works within the framework of the hospital and abides by its rules and regulations. The registered nurse has the responsibility for the nursing care of the patient. The practical nurse works under the supervision of the registered nurse and administers patient care. Both are directly responsible to their employer and are obligated to follow the policies of the hospital.

A hospital team (doctors, nurses, technicians, dietitians, social workers, and others) must work together toward a common goal if that goal is to be attained. A team whose spirit is high accomplishes much; a team whose spirit is low accomplishes very little. The patient suffers as a result of poor team spirit.

The patient's care is planned to ensure uniformity, which is vital to his recovery. The nursing care plan is a written, individualized course of action to meet the total needs of the patient. This specified method assists the patient in adjusting physically and emotionally to his condition. The following example will help to clarify the need for this written, individualized plan of action. A patient has his leg amputated and after full recovery has a prosthesis. On Monday a nurse enters the room and states, "I'm sorry your leg had to be amputated, Mr. Jones; I'll give you a bath to make it easier for you." In this instance the nurse expresses pity for the patient and makes him dependent. This is a poor approach because it delays the patient's progress and recovery by encouraging dependency. On Tuesday another nurse enters the room and remarks, "Mr. Jones, it's time for your morning bath. I'll bring you some warm water so that you can bathe yourself. I know that you can do this, but if you have any difficulty, I'll be glad to help you." At this point Mr. Jones must be thinking, "One nurse wants to do everything for me, while the second nurse wants me to do everything for myself. I wish they would get together so that I would know what they want me to do. One nurse feels sorry for me, while the other nurse accepts my condition." If Mr. Jones has a tendency to feel sorry for himself, he will dislike the second nurse, who failed to indulge him. The second nurse, however, is aware that the patient needs to accept his condition and help himself. A careful assessment and a well-written nursing care plan would help eliminate this type of situation because the plan would state a definite approach to be used by all nursing personnel.

Nursing assistants are also members of the health team. They are less skilled than you because of the amount of training they have had. They expect you to assist them in understanding and implementing the nursing care plan. When the plan is not followed and different approaches are used, which approach are they to follow? If you do not follow the physician's orders as written and use the same approach to the patient, how can the patient have confidence when he is feeling confused and insecure? You need to develop a respect for authority and manifest this in your conduct.

Another important characteristic of a good nurse is faith. Faith means confidence in yourself and in all those with whom you come into contact. Contacts may include members of the health team, patients, their families, or members of the community at large. You must believe in human goodness and recognize that all persons are created equal, regardless of color, race, or creed. As a nurse you must believe in your nursing vocation. It is one of the greatest, most satisfying, and most rewarding vocations available today. It is a valuable service to the community. With this faith the nursing profession will continue to advance and attract dedicated people to its service.

You must be willing to keep confidential any information learned or discovered through your care of the patient. Some facts are private and personal to the patient and are not to be discussed lightly with companions, the patient's family, your family, or outsiders. By disclosure of some information you may permanently damage the patient's reputation and future. You should listen attentively to the patient and to the things he tells you so that you can minister effectively to him. Your interest in his personal or past life is not to provide you with information about which to gossip. Your reputation or the patient's reputation may be at stake. The patient seeks your assistance to aid him in recovering physically, mentally, and emotionally. Any act that detracts from this goal is unethical and a violation of the patient's rights.

The patient's rights include the right to life, the right to be respected as an individual, the right to privacy, the right to grant or deny permission for medical and surgical procedures and to be used as a teaching or research subject, the right to know the physician who is directly responsible for his care, the right to know details of procedures and care prescribed and planned for his treatment, the right to know his diagnosis and prognosis, and the right to receive appropriate spiritual care.

In summary, the characteristics or qualities of a good nurse are dependability, knowledge, honesty, consideration, cheerfulness, and respect. As a practical nurse you must possess and manifest faith and integrity. You must respect the rights of others. If you become this type of person, you will be effective in your vocation as a practical nurse.

◆ *Study Helps*

1. Define the following:
   - Nursing
   - Practical nurse
   - Vocational nurse
   - Confidentiality
   - Hospital
   - Patient
   - Community
   - Peer
2. How does the practical nurse differ from the registered nurse?
3. Will the future of practical nursing change?
4. Which methods can you use to acquaint yourself with this new way of life?
5. List and explain the qualifications and abilities necessary for a practical nurse.

Bibliography

Brooke R, Tedrow MP, and Van Landingham J: Adaptation nursing practice, ed 1, St Louis, 1982, The CV Mosby Co.

Edelman C and Mandle CL: Health promotion throughout the lifespan, St Louis, 1986, The CV Mosby Co.

Harkness G and Dincher JR: Total patient care: foundations and practice, ed 7, St Louis, 1987, The CV Mosby Co.

Jacobson SF and McGrath HM: Nurses under stress, ed 1, New York, 1983, John Wiley & Sons, Inc.

Mechanic D: Handbook of health, health care and the health professions, ed 1, New York, 1983, Macmillan Co.

Stevens KR: Power and influence: a sourcebook for nurses, ed 1, New York, 1982, John Wiley & Sons, Inc.

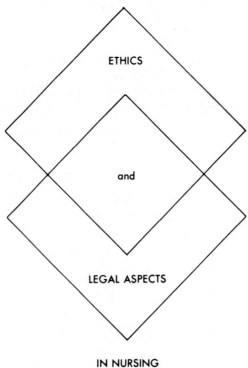

INTERRELATIONSHIP OF

ETHICS

and

LEGAL ASPECTS

IN NURSING

Influencing factors in nursing.

Objectives

At the completion of this chapter the student practical nurse will be able to:

◆ Define the practice of nursing as a practical nurse.

◆ List three patient rights as described in the Patient's Bill of Rights.

◆ List the requirements necessary to obtain licensure in the student's state of residence.

◆ Describe the legal duty the nurse owes to a patient.

◆ Name and describe two laws that govern the nurse's rights as an employee.

◆ State why the study of ethics is important for nurses.

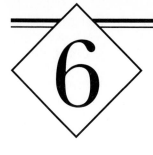

Code of Ethics and Legal Aspects of Nursing

Laura J. Reilly

◆ Ethics

Science and technology are developing at a rapid rate. At the same time, significant changes are occurring in the mores, values, and demographics of our society. Nurses are confronted by the evidence of the scientific and cultural changes almost daily: organ transplants, artificial organs, artificial respirators and other life-sustaining equipment, in vitro fertilization capability, the civil rights movement, the unionization of health care workers, human experimentation, an aging population, the rising cost of health care, a growing number of one-parent families, increasing numbers of homeless, a high incidence of teenage pregnancy, drug abuse, AIDS, suicide, and legalized abortion are but a few examples. Nurses will be faced with the many issues generated by these and other changes in their personal lives and in their profession.

Nurses make judgments in providing care for their patients. These judgments and actions may be required in a situation where the best interests of the patient or the family are not clear, as when the patient or the family refuses further medical or nursing care. The nurse may be confronted with a situation in which the patient's values conflict with the nurse's personal values, for example, when a nurse who believes abortion to be immoral is asked to care for a patient who is going to have or has had an abortion. The nurse may also experience conflicts with other health professionals regarding patient care.

How does the nurse cope with the technological and cultural changes and the conflicts that these changes and that everyday nursing practice present? What mainstay does the nurse rely on in making decisions and taking action? The nurse must have some guide to use especially in new or difficult situations. Ethics is the branch of philosophy that deals with questions of human conduct in situations where a decision must be made regarding what ought to be done or what is morally correct. Situations where there may be doubt as to the proper behavior or actions are called ethical dilemmas. These dilemmas often involve choices between equal unsatisfactory alternatives, situations with no apparent solutions, or interrelationships with conflict and tension.

Nurses need to examine their own individual values and ethics as part of the continuing process of maturing as both a person and as a professional. Knowing yourself is the first part of ethical development. The following types of questions are starting points in self-examination: What makes humans different from other animals? What is life? Has this definition changed within the last 10 years? What rights do minors or students have? What rights do patients have? What rights do human beings have? Do the rights of students, minors, patients, and humans differ? Is a person justified in taking an action because she "meant well?" What does freedom mean? What duties does a person have to others? What are characteristics of maturity? How do you respond when confronted by someone whose values are different from your own?

The individual who undertakes an action in a situation involving ethical choices has experienced, consciously or not, four phases: moral sensitivity, reasoning, motivation, and moral courage. Moral sensitivity is a recognition that the needs of another person exist and that you can have an impact on these needs. Nurses are trained to recognize people's needs so their moral sensitivity should be more developed. In the reasoning phase the individual examines the facts and the alternative actions and tries to determine which action is "right." In the motivation phase an individual's own self-interest becomes a factor. How will this action affect my career? What will others think of me? Can I afford to do this? Finally, moral courage is required for one to take the desirable action. A professional such as a nurse is supposed to embody the highest standards of society, but it is not always easy for the individual.

How do you overcome your fears and take action based on these standards and your conviction? Continuing education is one way that the professional is able to maintain a clear picture of the highest professional standards. Facing one's fear of isolation from peers or the fear of being branded a self-righteous person is also helpful. Discussions with others on these issues and critical thinking about how these issues and actions will be viewed 40 or 50 years from now also put these matters into a better perspective. The opinions of your peers today on an action taken based on moral judgments, for example, are not going to be very significant when you are 70 years old. The moral action will stand by itself when put into this perspective.

The development of an ethical leadership role requires focusing on what good an individual and his group can accomplish together, whether at work, home, or in the community. This requires a sensitivity to issues and a vision of what the group should be doing to address a particular issue. A group's attention to the needs of the homeless is an example of the result of someone's ethical leadership.

Professions have developed codes of ethics to serve as a guide for the professional's behavior and to give the public an indication as to the behavior that should be expected from a professional.

◆ The Code for Licensed Practical/Vocational Nurses

The National Federation of Licensed Practical Nurses (NFLPN) has adopted such a code of ethics. Each LPN is expected to adhere to the standards of practice and conducts set forth in this Code of Ethics, as amended in 1979.

1. Know the scope of maximum utilization of the LPN/VN and function within the scope.
2. Recognize and appreciate cultural backgrounds and spiritual needs, respecting the religious belief of individual patients.
3. Safeguard the confidential information acquired from any source about the patient.
4. Refuse to give endorsement to the sale and promotion of commercial products or services.
5. Uphold the high standards and personal appearance, language, dress, and demeanor.
6. Accept responsibility of membership in NFLPN and participate in its efforts to maintain the established standards of nursing practice and employment policies conducive to quality patient care.

◆ Standards

In 1979, the NFLPN adopted standards for nursing practice. These provide a model for the profession to assist in ensuring the provision of quality nursing care.

I. Education
   A. Shall complete a formal education program in practical nursing approved by the appropriate nursing authority in a state
   B. Shall participate in initial orientation within the employing institution.

II. Legal/ethical status
   A. Shall hold a current license to practice nursing as an LP/VN in accordance with the law of the state wherein employed
   B. Shall know the scope of nursing practice authorized by the Nurse Practice Act in the state wherein employed
   C. Shall have a personal commitment to fulfill the legal responsibilities inherent in good nursing practice
   D. Shall take responsible actions in situations wherein there is unprofessional conduct by a health care provider
   E. Shall recognize and have a commitment to meet the ethical and moral obligations of the practice of nursing

III. Practice
   A. Shall accept assigned responsibilities as an accountable member of the health care team
   B. Shall function within the limits of educational preparation and experience as related to the assigned duties
   C. Shall function with other members of the health care team in promoting and maintaining health, preventing disease and disability, caring

for and rehabilitating individuals who are experiencing altered health state

D. Shall know and utilize the nursing process in planning, implementing, and evaluating health services and nursing care to the individual patient or group

   1. Planning: The planning of nursing includes:
   - a. Assessment of health status of the individual patient, the family, and community groups
   - b. An analysis of the information gained from assessment
   - c. The identification of health goals

   2. Implementation: The plan for nursing care is implemented to achieve the stated goals:
   - a. Observing, recording, and reporting significant changes which require intervention or different goals
   - b. Applying nursing knowledge and skills to promote and maintain health, prevent disease and disability, and optimize functional capabilities of an individual patient
   - c. Assisting the patient and family with activities of daily living and encouraging self-care as appropriate
   - d. Carrying out therapeutic regimens prescribed by a physician or other authorized health care providers

   3. Evaluation: The plan for nursing care and its implementation are evaluated to measure the progress toward the stated goals and will include appropriate persons and/or groups to determine:
   - a. The relevancy of current goals, in relation to the progress of the individual patient, the family, and community
   - b. The involvement of the recipients of care in the evaluation process
   - c. The quality of the nursing action in the implementation of the plan
   - d. A reordering of priorities or new goal setting in the care plan

E. Shall participate in peer review and other evaluative processes

F. Shall participate in the development of policies concerning the health and nursing needs of society and in the roles and functions of the LP/VN

IV. Continuing education

A. Shall be responsible for maintaining the highest possible level of professional competence at all times

B. Shall periodically reassess career goals and select continuing education activities which will help to achieve these goals

C. Shall take advantage of continuing education opportunities, which will lead to personal growth and professional development including: reading new publications and periodicals; self-study programs; membership in their professional organization; seminars and community health activities

D. Shall seek and participate in formal continuing education activities which are measurable such as the nationally accepted and recognized CEU

These standards recognize the need for nurses to have a sound ethical basis.

An examination of the principles that underlie ethical actions in nursing would also be helpful to nurses in establishing a basis on which to formulate judgments and actions. One author has suggested the following principles, which, although not exhaustive, are appropriate for consideration by nurses as a foundation for their actions. These include:

1. The principle of respect for individuals as persons. This includes a respect for the individual as a unique, autonomous individual whose values and goals require consideration, whose value is equal to every other individual, and who also, as a person, has responsibilities and obligations to others as a member of a community.

2. The principle of beneficence. This principle requires the nurse to be thoughtful and take action that minimizes possible harm and promotes the benefit and well-being of others in a given situation. This may, of course, require the balancing of harms versus benefits in order to promote health. The nurse who is considerate, for example, may have to weigh the psychological harm of using physical restraints on an elderly, confused or sedated patient against the benefit of preventing this patient from harming himself by getting out of bed unattended.

3. The principle of justice requires fairness in the treatment of patients.

◆ A Patient's Bill of Rights

Consideration of the rights of others in developing an ethical basis for nursing practices has become especially important in recent years with the consumer movement. Health consumers are increasingly aware of their rights to health care and their rights to make decisions regarding their health care. Rights of groups or individuals usually denote duties or responsibilities of those who come into contact with the individuals or groups. In 1973 the American Hospital Association declared the following Patient's Bill of Rights. The nurse should be aware of these rights when planning and giving nursing care.

1. The patient has the right to considerate and respectful care.

2. The patient has the right to obtain from his physician complete current information concerning his diagnosis, treatment, and prognosis, in terms the patient can be reasonably expected to understand. When it is not medically advisable to give such information to the patient, the information should be made available to an appropriate person in his behalf. He has the right to know by name the physician responsible for coordinating his care.

3. The patient has the right to receive from his physician information necessary to give informed consent prior to the start of any procedure and/or treatment. Except in emergencies, such information for informed consent should include, but not necessarily be limited to, the specific procedure and/or treatment, the medically significant risks involved, and the probable duration of incapacitation. Where medically significant alternatives for care or treatment exist, or when the patient requests information concerning medical

alternatives, the patient has the right to such information. The patient also has the right to know the name of the person responsible for the procedures and/or treatment.

4. The patient has the right to refuse treatment to the extent permitted by law and to be informed of the medical consequences of his action.

5. The patient has the right to every consideration of his privacy concerning his own medical care program. Case discussion, consultation, examination, and treatment are confidential and should be conducted discreetly. Those not directly involved in his care must have the permission of the patient to be present.

6. The patient has the right to expect that all communications and records pertaining to his care should be treated as confidential.

7. The patient has the right to expect that within its capacity a hospital must make reasonable response to the request of a patient for services. The hospital must provide evaluation, service, and/or referral as indicated by the urgency of the case. When medically permissible, a patient may be transferred to another facility only after he has received complete information and explanation concerning the needs for and alternatives to such a transfer. The institution to which the patient is transferred must first have accepted the patient for transfer.

8. The patient has the right to obtain information as to any relationship of his hospital to other health care and educational institutions insofar as his care is concerned. The patient has the right to obtain information as to the existence of any professional relationships among individuals, by name, who are treating him.

9. The patient has the right to be advised if the hospital proposes to engage in or perform human experimentation affecting his care or treatment. The patient has the right to refuse to participate in such research projects.

10. The patient has the right to expect reasonable continuity of care. He has the right to know in advance what appointment times and physicians are available and where. The patient has the right to expect that the hospital will provide a mechanism whereby he is informed by this physician or a delegate of the physician of the patient's continuing health.

11. The patient has the right to examine and receive an explanation of his bill regardless of source of payment.

12. The patient has the right to know what hospital rules and regulations apply to his conduct as a patient.

Although the Patient's Bill of Rights, in many respects, is directed toward physicians and hospitals, it has clear implications for nurses. The nurse is usually with the patient more frequently than anyone else on the health care team. It is the nurse who often first learns that the patient desires certain information or does not understand the treatment program that has been prescribed by the physician. The nurse should communicate this information to the appropriate professional. This is but one example of how the nurse can assist patients in obtaining full realization of their rights as a patient. Other portions of the Patient's Bill of Rights have direct implications for nurses as, for example, the patient's right to reasonable continuity of care, right to privacy, and right to a reasonable response to a request for services. Examination of the Patient's Bill of Rights should assist the nurse in becoming more empathetic to the patient's needs and rights.

The nurse will be faced with many ethical dilemmas throughout his or her career requiring that all available resources be used, including personal and professional ethical guides, peers, educators, supervisors, clergy, and professional associations to assist the nurse in recognizing, discussing, and arriving at a course of conduct that is respectful of the patient, responsible, just, and one with which the nurse can live.

◆ The Nurse and the Public

Nurses are expected to be accountable for their judgments and actions in caring for patients. That is, nurses answer to patients and society as a whole in courts of law for violation of the patient's rights or neglect of the nurse's duty to the patient. Therefore in addition to reliance on ethical conduct, nurses must also be familiar with the legal standards governing nursing practice.

Nursing Practice Acts

All states have nursing practice acts that, in general, state a definition of nursing, outline the requirements for licensure, establish a board of nursing to implement the law, provide for suspension or revocation of the license under certain conditions, and establish penalties for practicing nursing without a license.

The definition of a licensed practical nurse, which varies from state to state, has become very important to nurses in recent years as the practical nursing role expands and practical nurses desire a more accurate description of their profession. Nurses are concerned that the legal definition encompass the entire scope or range of nursing activities to ensure that the nurse performing such activities will not be practicing outside the legally defined scope. The nurse who does practice outside the legal definition of nursing risks civil liability, criminal penalties or both.

The statutory definition of licensed practical nursing in the New Jersey Nurse Practice Act is an example of one definition that has been revised within the past decade in recognition of the need licensed practical nurses have for a more comprehensive definition. The New Jersey definition now states:

> The practice of nursing as a licensed practical nurse is defined as performing tasks and responsibilities within the framework of casefinding; reinforcing the patient and family teaching program through health teaching, health counseling and provision of supportive and restorative care, under the direction of a registered nurse or licensed or otherwise legally authorized physician or dentist.*

The licensed practical nurse should be familiar with the statutory definition of practical nursing of the state in which the nurse is practicing. This will facilitate the recognition of any possible conflicts between the legally defined scope of practical

---

*From New Jersey Statutes Annotated, vol. 45, pp. 11-23.

nursing practice and the actual tasks and functions the licensed practical nurse is performing. If the practical nurse recognizes a possible conflict, assistance from the nurse's employer, the nurse's professional association, and, if necessary, an attorney should be sought. Until resolution of the existence of a conflict or an actual conflict is reached, the nurse should be relieved of the duties that are the subject of the conflict.

State Boards of Nursing

Nurse practice acts provide for the establishment of state boards of nursing. These are independent agencies of the state government charged with implementing the laws that regulate the practice of nursing within the state. The governor of the state usually appoints members of the state board of nursing. Membership on the board may consist of nurses only or may include physicians, hospital administrators, and members of the general public. The latter members represent the consumer's interest in the provision of quality nursing care. The state board of nursing governs both registered nurses and licensed practical nurses in all but eight states. These eight states have separate boards of nursing to administer the laws for licensed practical nurses.

General activities of the state boards of nursing include (1) the establishment of minimum criteria for approval of nursing schools; (2) the approval of schools of nursing that meet the established criteria, and the denial or withdrawal of approval from schools that fail to meet these requirements; (3) the examination of applicants for licensure to practice; (4) the issuance of licenses to qualified applicants; (5) the investigation of violations of the nursing practice act; (6) the investigation of any charges of unsafe or incompetent nursing actions; and (7) the denial, suspension, or revocation of a license for an established cause.

Licensure

Licensure is the process by which a government agency grants permission to persons to engage in a given profession or occupation by certifying that those who are licensed have attained the minimum degree of competency necessary to ensure that the public health, safety, and welfare will be protected. Licensure is provided for by the nursing practice acts of the states. Almost all of these laws are mandatory and require that everyone who practices nursing for compensation must be licensed. The only exceptions to this mandatory requirement are student nurses, employees of the federal government licensed in another state, and those involved in emergency situations.

The requirements that an applicant must meet to obtain licensure vary from state to state. In general the applicant must (1) have completed a minimum of 2 years of high school or its equivalent, (2) have completed an approved educational program in practical nursing, and (3) be a U.S. citizen or have a current visa. If these requirements are met, the applicant must then pass an examination. If the applicant passes, the license is granted.

The current examination being used is the National Council Licensing Examination for Practical Nursing (NCLEX-PN). Appendix C provides information about the NCLEX-PN test and helpful tips for taking the examination. This examination was started in 1985 and is being used for practical nurse licensure in all states except California. The examination is given twice a year in April and October on the same day in every state. The examination consists of approximately 250 multiple choice questions. It is a 1-day examination. A minimum score of 350 is required to qualify for licensure. The practical nurse is notified of a pass or fail grade; however, the numerical score is not included. If the applicant passes the examination, a license is granted. If the applicant fails the examination, a detailed diagnostic profile is sent to the nurse identifying the areas to review before retesting. Permission must usually be obtained to take the examination again at the next scheduled examination date. Some states require that additional courses of study be completed before repeating the examination. It should be noted that fulfillment of the minimal requirements for licensure does not indicate that *good* nursing care will be provided by the licensee; the licensure procedure is only an attempt by the state to ensure that the licensee is capable of providing *safe* nursing care.

State laws or regulations provide for some exceptions to the preceding procedure for obtaining a nursing license. These regulations allow licensure of applicants who are already registered in another state. The procedures include endorsement and waiver.

Licensure by endorsement occurs when a state board of nursing reviews the application of a nurse who is licensed in another state to determine whether the nurse's qualifications were equivalent to their own requirements at the time the nurse was first licensed. It usually requires that the examinations of the two states were comparable at that time and that the applicant's score on the examination would have been a passing score in both states. Endorsement has been simplified in most states by the development of national nursing examinations.

Licensure by waiver occurs if the applicant does not meet all the specific requirements for licensure but has qualifications that are equivalent. The specific requirements for education, experience, or examination may then be waived by the state board of nursing. Other states require that all out-of-state nurses pass the regular examination to obtain licensure. Licensure by endorsement or waiver is not as common as by examination.

Suspension or Revocation

State boards of nursing have the power to suspend or revoke a nurse's license. This power enables state boards to protect the patient and the profession from unfit and incompetent nurses. The reasons for which a state board may suspend or revoke a license usually include:

1. Fraud or willful misrepresentation in procuring a license as a practical nurse
2. Conviction of a felony (a serious crime)
3. Drug abuse or addiction
4. Mental or physical incompetency
5. Unprofessional or dishonorable conduct
6. Dishonesty
7. Provision of unsafe or incompetent nursing care
8. Violation of provisions of the nursing practice act

Before the state board can suspend or revoke a nurse's license, the board must notify the nurse of the charges and provide an opportunity for a hearing. At the hearing the nurse or the nurse's attorney will be allowed to question any witnesses and present evidence in the nurse's defense.

Renewal

Once a license is obtained, it must be renewed periodically. In some states, the license must be renewed every year, whereas other states provide that it must be renewed every other year. In most states the failure to renew a license at the designated time results in automatic placement on the inactive list. While a nurse is on the inactive list, the nurse will not have to pay renewal fees but cannot practice nursing. If the nurse wants to become active as a licensed practical nurse again, an application for reinstatement should be completed. In addition, a reinstatement fee is usually required.

In at least nine states, to renew the license nurses must present evidence to the state licensure board of attendance in continuing education programs. This is an attempt to ensure that nurses will remain competent in their practice by learning new techniques, new approaches to patient care, and other developments in health care and nursing. In some instances, it is up to the nurse to maintain the documentation of attendance at approved continuing legal education activities. It should be noted that in many instances only certain types of programs, which have been previously approved, will be accepted to meet the requirements for renewal. Therefore if there are any questions about the educational requirements for renewal, the questions should be directed to the specific board of the state in which the nurse has licensure.

◆ The Nurse's Relationship With the Patient

Torts

Tort is the French synonym for the English word *wrong*. A tort is a wrongful act or failure to act that causes injury to another person or his property. The act or failure to act is a breach of a duty owed to another or the invasion of a legally protected right of another. The person who commits a tort may be held civilly liable to the injured person and will usually have to pay money to compensate the victim for the injuries. It differs from a crime, which is an offense against society as well as against the injured person. A crime is punishable by a fine paid to the state and/or imprisonment rather than by money damages paid to the victim.

There are many types of torts. The following torts are only those with which the licensed practical nurse would most commonly be concerned.

Negligence and malpractice. *Negligence* is the failure of a person to exercise the degree of care that an ordinarily prudent person would exercise in similar circumstances to prevent injury to another person or his property. It is negligence only if the person who causes the injury owes a legal duty to exercise care to the person who is injured.

It should be noted that if the negligent act is such a flagrant and reckless disregard for the safety of another that it endangers that person's life, the act may be one of criminal negligence and be subject to criminal penalties and civil liability.

Malpractice, a form of negligence, is the term used when a professional, such as a nurse or a physician, does not have or does not use the skills and knowledge commonly possessed by other members of the profession and thereby causes harm to a patient. For malpractice to occur, the nurse need not intend to harm the patient. A licensed practical nurse is held to a higher standard than the ordinarily prudent person because of the competencies the nurse professes to possess. The licensed practical nurse must have and use the knowledge and skills required of the licensed practical nurse. When the nurse is using the skills and training of the profession, this higher standard of care applies.

The legal duty of a nurse arises from the relationship between the nurse and the patient. Every nurse owes a patient the duty to exercise the care of an ordinarily prudent nurse to prevent injury to the patient. If the nurse meets the level of performance that the ordinarily prudent licensed practical nurse with equivalent skills and training would have met in the same situation, negligence has not occurred; instead an unavoidable incident has occurred, and the nurse is not liable for any resulting injuries. Thus a licensed practical nurse who fills a hot water bottle with excessively hot water and places it against the skin of an unconscious patient where it causes a burn would be liable for negligence. The ordinarily prudent licensed practical nurse would have exercised care to see that the water was the correct temperature and would not have caused this injury to the patient. Other acts of negligence that are frequently the subjects of malpractice lawsuits when an injury results are the failure to prevent a patient from falling, especially if the patient is elderly, sedated, suffers from dizziness, or has a visual problem; administration of the wrong medication or wrong dosage of medication; failure to verify a physician's order when it is not legible or not understood; failure to observe and evaluate a patient's condition, such as the circulation in a leg that has been placed in a cast; failure to report a known condition to the appropriate person, such as failure to report to the surgeon the observation of a patient's inability to urinate before surgery; and the nurse's failure to stay with a patient until it is safe or prudent to leave.

Several decisions make it clear that nurses are required, under certain circumstances, to exercise independent professional judgment and that failure to do so may result in the nurse's being held liable to the patient for the damages the patient suffered, independently or separately from a determination of whether a physician or hospital is also liable. Formerly nurses were able to avoid or minimize their liability by shifting their legal responsibility to the physician or hospital under legal theories such as *respondeat superior,* the borrowed servant, charitable immunity, or the "captain of the ship" doctrine. More recently decisions verify that the nurse is held to the standard of an independent professional responsible for her actions regardless of whether the physician or hospital are to be held liable also.

One doctrine or rule of law that may be raised by the plaintiff in a lawsuit based on malpractice is known as *res ipsa loquitur.* Literally this means "the thing speaks for itself." If the injury was the type that does not usually occur unless there is negligence, if the conduct or instrument causing the injury was in the exclusive control of the defendant, and if the injured person did not contribute to the negligence that caused the injury, this rule will be applied. That is, it is used when the defendant is in control of all possible causes of the injury and is better able to give evidence of what caused the injury. If all of the factors are present and the doctrine is applied, the defendant will be held liable for negligence. An example of a lawsuit where the rule was applied involved a patient who sustained serious injuries to an arm during an appendectomy.

If a nurse is sued for negligence or malpractice by a patient, the nurse can assert the defense that she acted as an ordinarily prudent nurse or that her actions did not cause the injury. In addition, the nurse can raise the defenses of contributory negligence, comparative negligence, or assumption of risk, if applicable.

Contributory negligence is unreasonable conduct by the patient that contributes to cause the injury. In this case the patient will not be able to recover compensation for his injuries. In the example of the excessively hot water bottle placed by the nurse, a patient who was conscious would have had a duty to take reasonable care to protect himself from harm. Failure to complain about the excessive heat might be deemed to constitute contributory negligence.

Under the *comparative negligence* statutes enacted by a few states, if both parties, the plaintiff and defendant, have contributed to the cause of the injury, the negligence is apportioned between the two parties, and the plaintiff is allowed to recover only to the extent that the defendant caused the injury. If the defendant, for example, is found to have contributed 75% of the negligence that caused the plaintiff's injury and the total damages to the plaintiff are deemed to be worth $10,000, the plaintiff would be awarded only $7500. Under some comparative negligence statutes the plaintiff must have contributed less than half (50%) of the negligence that caused the injury, or he will be barred from receiving any money damages from the defendant.

The *assumption of risk* defense asserts that the patient knew the risk attached to actions the nurse was about to do or not do and the patient voluntarily consented to them and thereby assumed the risk of the resulting injury. This defense might be used if a patient voluntarily consented to take an investigational drug after being informed of all the risks it presented.

Another defense may be available to the licensed practical nurse who is sued when the nursing care was rendered at the scene of an accident. Statutes or laws known as "Good Samaritan statutes" have been enacted by legislatures in most states. These laws encourage health professionals to stop and give assistance to accident victims by limiting the liability of the professional to injuries caused by gross negligence and intentionally harmful acts provided that the professional gives the care in good faith and in the belief that the circumstances constituted an actual emergency. Gross negligence is flagrant carelessness and would require the plaintiff in a lawsuit to prove that the licensed practical nurse not only did not act as a reasonably prudent licensed practical nurse would have at the scene of the accident but also that the practical nurse (defendant) acted with flagrant disregard for the patient.

Malpractice lawsuits became a growing concern for health care personnel during the 1970s. Because of a new emphasis on consumer rights, greater public understanding of the standards of health care the patient should receive, and a lack of personalized health care, the number of lawsuits mushroomed. In a lawsuit the "shotgun" approach is used to ensure that the party who was ultimately responsible for the patient's alleged injury is named as a defendant. That is, anyone who could possibly be responsible and be liable for a money judgment is named as a defendant, including the physician, the hospital, and the nurse. It can be expensive and emotionally traumatic for the nurse to defend herself and show that the responsibility, if any, for the patient's alleged injury lies elsewhere. Therefore prevention of malpractice litigation is everyone's concern, including the nurse's. Of course the consistent provision of good nursing care is one of the nurse's strongest safeguards. Maintaining friendly but professional relationships with patients is also a preventive measure. The patient will feel that someone does care about what is happening to him. This is especially helpful if the patient is "suit prone." A suit-prone patient is insecure and demonstrates it by being resentful, uncooperative, and dissatisfied. This patient copes with his feelings of inadequacy by attempting to put others in a position of being at fault or blaming them for anything he perceives as wrong with his life. Particular attention should be paid to this patient's psychological needs. Another preventive measure is the maintenance of good medical records. If the patient who perceives his care as being unsatisfactory or negligent seeks an attorney, one of the attorney's first actions after interviewing the patient is to review the medical record. If the medical record is complete and provides a clear description of the patient's care, the attorney may find that the care was competent and thorough and so advise the patient. The attorney will not need to file a lawsuit to ascertain the source of the patient's alleged injuries because the record is complete.

Breach of contract. The relationship between nurses and institutions such as hospitals and the relationship between nurses and patients are based on a contract or agreement. The contract does not have to be written on paper to exist. A nurse breaches this contract with the institution when the nurse fails to provide services that have been agreed on orally or in writing or by failing to provide services usually or customarily provided by a nurse or reasonably expected by a patient.

Assault and battery. *Assault* is an intentional threat by one person to inflict injury or use unlawful physical force on another that creates an apprehension of imminent danger in the person who is threatened. *Battery* is the actual infliction of physical force or injury on another person. It is an unlawful touching of someone. The nurse who threatens a patient unjustifiably with the use of physical restraints is committing an assault. Liability for battery usually involves instances of failure to obtain a patient's consent for a treatment or surgery. The legal right of a patient to determine what shall be done to his body is recognized throughout the United States. A doctrine of informed consent has developed based on this right through case law written by courts. Informed consent requires more than a patient's signature on a surgical or treatment consent form. It requires that the patient must receive an adequate explanation by the physician with details usually given by another physician in the same situation or one that gives the patient enough information, in understandable language, so that a reasonable person in the circumstances could make an intelligent decision regarding the proposed treatment. The explanation must include the necessity for the treatment, the risks attendant to the treatment, the desired outcome of the treatment, alternative treatments that are reasonably available, the consequences of foregoing the treatment, and any other information that would be helpful to the patient regarding the performance of the treatment or its effects. The nurse's role in obtaining informed consent is usually that of a witness to the discussion of a proposed treatment between the physician and patient and of the signature obtained on a consent form. The practical nurse should be alert for signs that the patient does not comprehend what has been said or written and communicate this to the physician. If the nurse serves as a witness, the nurse should note the circumstances of the consent in the patient's medical chart, including the patient's mental status. The patient must be alert and not medicated with sedatives or other drugs that cause confusion so he can give a knowing, willing, valid consent. Only in emergency situations, when the procedure is necessary to save the patient's life or prevent irreparable damage, is it unnecessary to obtain the patient's consent. In these cases the law implies or gives the patient's consent for him.

False imprisonment. *False imprisonment* is the unlawful restraint on the freedom of a person or an unlawful detention of a person. Physical force is not necessary. Words or threats that create a fear that force will be used to detain the person constitute false imprisonment. An example of false imprisonment is a nurse's retention of a person for failure to pay the hospital bill by locking the patient's door.

A situation that commonly arises involves the patient who is of sound mind and desires to leave the hospital although the physician and nurse believe he needs further care. The patient should be allowed to leave. However, before the patient leaves, the nature of his condition and the reasons he should stay in the hospital for additional care, as well as any possible consequences of leaving, should be explained to the patient. The patient should then be asked to sign a form that releases the hospital from liability for any of these consequences. Additionally, the nurse should note in the chart the patient's insistence on leaving and the explanation, or attempted explanation, to the patient of the consequences of leaving.

The charge of false imprisonment as well as battery may arise if physical restraints are used on a patient. Such restraints should be used with care and only when it is reasonable to do so for the patient's safety and welfare if less restrictive alternatives are not available. Today the use of tranquilizing drugs, if appropriate, makes the use of such restraints less common.

Invasion of privacy. The *right of privacy* is the right of a person to be free from unwarranted and unwanted exposure or publicity, that is, the right to not have one's body, name, picture, or *private* affairs exposed or made public without consent. The information contained in a patient's chart is confidential, as is the information that the patient communicates to the nurse. In some states this communication is protected by privilege statutes that prevent the disclosure of information obtained during the course of evaluation and treatment of the patient. Additionally, case law defining the right of privacy prevents disclosure of information obtained during the course of the patient's treatment and information that would harm the patient's reputation, business, or livelihood. Thus a nurse has a legal and an even broader ethical duty not to disclose information regarding the patient unless the patient expressly waives his right of privacy. The right of privacy also mandates that a nurse should not permit a photograph to be taken of the patient without the written permission of the patient or the patient's guardian.

The nurse must protect the patient from unwanted or unwarranted exposure to others. The patient has a right to be seen and examined only by those who are actually caring for him or those to whom the patient has given permission. This right exists in the hospital corridors, treatment rooms, and the patient's room. The nurse should protect the patient by covering the patient, drawing curtains, and closing doors when necessary to prevent the patient from being exposed to visitors, roommates, or hospital personnel.

There are some exceptions to the patient's right to privacy. A person cannot complain when facts that are a matter of public record, open to public inspection, or engaged in before the public are given publicity. These are public facts not private facts. Public facts would include a marriage or birthdate or the occupation in which the person publicly engages. Another exception pertains to public figures. A public figure is a person who seeks public recognition, such as a politician, author, or actor. Almost anything a public figure does is of legitimate interest to the public and therefore is not private. Still another exception exists under statutes that recognize that the preservation of public health outweighs the individual's right to privacy. These statutes require disclosure of certain facts by health professionals such as child abuse–reporting statutes, communicable disease–reporting statutes, and those statutes requiring report of any gunshot wounds.

A number of states are addressing the issue of whether confidential medical information concerning an individual with a contagious or communicable disease must be disclosed even against the wishes of the patient. In the past a person with a venereal disease, for example, has been subject to such involuntary disclosure. AIDS has prompted a reexamination of this issue, with arguments being made for and against disclosure of the condition. Laws of individual states should be consulted regarding this issue.

Defamation. *Defamation* is injury to the reputation and character of another person through false and malicious statements to a third person. *Libel* is a written statement, whereas *slander* is an oral statement. It would be a breach of a legal and ethical relationship with the patient for a nurse to talk about a patient in such a way that would expose him to public hatred, contempt, or ridicule. Additionally, any slander that alleges that the patient is (1) guilty of committing a crime that can be characterized as vile or depraved, (2) alleges that the patient has a venereal disease, (3) alleges that the patient is incompetent in his business or profession, or (4) alleges that the patient is unchaste is considered to be damaging *per se*. Slander of these four types is the basis for awarding a plaintiff money without the plaintiff needing to prove that he was actually injured by such slander.

In addition to tortious liability, the nurse's relationship with the patient entails certain other responsibilities.

Medical Records

The patient's chart contains all information regarding the care and treatment given to the patient. It is the means by which the members of the health team and consultants communicate so that all information is shared. This ensures that the patient's care is complete and important information is not misplaced, forgotten, or lost. It is also used for research and evaluation of the care patients are receiving.

The patient's chart is a legal document and may be used in a courtroom as evidence of the care the patient received. The hospital can be held liable for failure to maintain accurate records. The nurse's continual contact with a patient puts the nurse in the best position to observe the patient's condition as well as treatments and medications that the patient receives. These observations should be written in the patient's chart.

When the nurse is charting, it is important to ensure that:

1. The chart is legible
2. The chart is complete, accurate, and factual
3. The chart is written in ink without any erasures (Errors should be crossed through with the nurse's signature or initials above or beside the error along with the date and time the error is noted.)
4. The chart includes the date, time, and patient's name on each sheet
5. Spelling and abbreviations are correct
6. Visits by physicians, consultants, and supervisors are recorded
7. The use of statements that are merely hearsay or gossip is avoided

For purposes of accuracy and completeness the nurse's notes should include specific observations (not general descriptions) of the following:

1. The type, frequency, and any difficulty encountered in giving nursing care
2. The response of the patient to the nursing and medical care
3. The condition of the patient as observed periodically by the nurse
4. The degree of cooperativeness or hostility demonstrated by the patient
5. Symptoms, signs, and actions demonstrated by the patient and any changes in these
6. The mental attitude of the patient, including any complaints
7. Procedures and medication, including the routes and times they are given
8. All reactions to medications and treatments
9. The patient's signature of any legal documents including a notation of anyone with the patient and the patient's condition

The nurse's notes should be signed by the nurse at the end of each entry. The signature should be written and should include the first name or initial, last name in full, and the nurse's title.

Medications

Aside from the practical nurse's obligation to administer medications safely to patients, the nurse should be aware of state and federal laws governing drugs. Violation of these laws may be grounds for severe censure, suspension, or revocation of the nurse's license.

The Drug Abuse Prevention and Control Act is the federal statute that governs the permissible distribution of controlled substances. Controlled substances that are specified by this statute include narcotics, hallucinogenic drugs, and barbiturates. The statute separates these drugs into five schedules or categories according to their potential for abuse, their usefulness for medical treatment, and whether use of the drug leads to physiological and psychological dependence. Some of the regulations differ according to the schedule the drug is in, but in general, all prescriptions for controlled substances must be dated and signed by the physician or dentist and must have the patient's full name and address. The prescription must also have the name, address, and registration number of the prescribing physician or dentist.

The nurse may administer to the patient the individual dosage prescribed by a written order. This is the only lawful use that a nurse may make of a controlled substance. All controlled substances that have been prescribed for patients must be stored securely to prevent loss or theft. Complete and accurate inventory records must be kept of all controlled substances received at the nurses' station and administered to patients.

States also regulate the dispensing and administration of drugs. Most states have their own version of the controlled substances act, which includes prescription and inventory requirements. Additionally, the states have pharmacy acts that prohibit anyone but a licensed pharmacist or other exempted persons from preparing, dispensing, retailing, and administering drugs, medicines, or chemicals. A physician is exempt when these acts are done in the treatment of patients in the physician's medical practice. A nurse is exempt only when administering a medicine to a patient under the written or oral prescription of a physician or dentist.

Death

Medicine and nursing are usually devoted to sustaining life and promoting recovery. Death, however, is inevitable for everyone and a frequent occurrence in health care settings. With the development and use of life-sustaining respirators and other equipment, death is no longer a precise concept, from either an ethical or legal perspective. At the same time, the ability to transplant organs from one person to another has complicated the legal considerations of death because the law desires to protect the dying individual who may be a prospective organ donor while recognizing the beneficent purposes such transplants serve. Traditionally, death meant the permanent cessation of respiration, circulation, and pulsation without hope of resuscitation. Today, in addition to the traditional view, the definition of death is being expanded to include brain death as measured by electronic equipment. At least six states have by statute defined death with this alternative definition.

Euthanasia, literally translated, means "good death," but is usually interpreted by the public to mean "mercy killing." Euthanasia is usually subdivided into active and passive euthanasia. Active euthanasia involves an affirmative, intentional act to shorten or terminate the life of a terminally ill patient. It is voluntary if the terminally ill patient asks another to do the act; otherwise it is involuntary. Passive euthanasia, the omission or failure to give a lifesaving or life-supporting treatment to a patient, may also be voluntary if requested by the patient. This is not uncommon as more patients seek death with dignity and assert their rights to refuse unwanted medical or nursing care.

Terminally ill persons have been given judicially recognized rights, within limits, to end their lives by refusing continued medical treatment. The clear trend in court decisions is to place great importance on a patient's wishes when they are in conflict with their family's, doctor's, hospital's, church's, or community's values. Although the state has an interest in preserving life, a person's right to govern oneself and one's affairs is valued also. The courts are also recognizing the right of family members to make this decision when the patient is unable to make the decision because of a medical condition such as a permanent comatose state.

Active euthanasia, however, could subject the nurse to both criminal and civil penalties. Although penalties could be imposed for an omission constituting passive euthanasia, at least where it is not protected by law, the probability of such sanctions is far less likely, especially when the omission is voluntary.

The nurse should accurately record any comments of the patient and of the patient's family regarding death and the use of extraordinary measures to sustain life of the terminally ill patient. Such notes may be helpful in supporting a patient or family in making and accepting a decision at a later time. Such notes can also be used if the family of a patient pursues a wrongful death action or a negligence lawsuit following the patient's death.

The ability of science and technology to prolong life has resulted in a drive for legislation in some states to allow people to plan ahead for the event of a terminal illness to prevent what the individual considers unnecessary prolongation of life because of a belief in the patient's right to die by what is popularly called a *living will*. The living will is signed by an individual when he is still rational and capable of considering the full implications of such a document. The living will instructs the physician or health care providers not to prolong life when recovery from a terminal illness cannot be expected. Laws such as that currently in place in New Mexico, NMSA, 1978, 24-7-1 to 24-7-11, for example, relieve the health care provider from liability for following the patient's wishes as stated in a living will. The formal requirements of a normal will (see below) must be met for the living will to be valid.

Wills

A will is the declaration of a person, who is called the *will maker* or *testator,* as to the settlement and to whom he wishes his property distributed after his death. It may also declare the person's wishes regarding the care of any minor children or other dependents. A will can save time and possibly taxes for the survivors. If there is no will, the property is distributed according to state law regardless of the deceased's actual wishes or the survivors' needs.

A will should be written by an attorney unless death is imminent to ensure compliance with laws of the various states. The nurse should assist the patient in contacting the patient's attorney. If the nurse is asked to witness the will, the nurse may do so but should realize that it could result in being called to testify in court at a later time if the will is contested. The nurse should not be a witness if receiving a bequest or gift under the terms of the will because it may negate the bequest.

By signing the will after the testator, the witness is saying that the testator's signature is genuine. The witness should be prepared to testify in court if the will is later contested. In addition, for a will to be valid the testator must be of sound mind. This means that the testator must understand that he is making a will, know the nature and extent of his property, and know the persons who would normally receive his property, such as the immediate family, if he desires to give it to someone else. Because a witness is present at the signing of the will, the witness may be called on to testify as to any observations about the testator that would support or refute the testator's mental capacity to make a will. The nurse who knows a patient is signing a will, whether or not the nurse is serving as a witness, should record the execution or making of the will along with any observations of the patient in the patient's chart.

◆ The Nurse as an Employee

Contracts

A *contract* is a promise or a set of promises between two or more persons that creates a legal relationship between them and a legal obligation that one or more of them must fulfill. The usual contract the licensed practical nurse will encounter is the employment contract. Although it is desirable to have a written employment contract, an oral employment contract may be binding on the nurse and the employer. Under the employment contract it is the nurse's obligation to perform nursing functions with the skills and knowledge of a licensed practical nurse in accordance with the standards of the profession and any additional qualifications the nurse represented he or she possessed to the employer. The employer has the duty to provide a safe working environment, sufficient and competent fellow workers, and safe equipment. Failure on the part of the nurse or the employer to perform these duties is a breach of the contract. A breach of a contract can result in a lawsuit to seek a court to order the breaching party to perform the obligations of the contract or to pay money to the party who was damaged by the breach. However, a nurse will usually not be required to perform if she refuses to work for the employer because the contract is one for personal services. Rather, the nurse might be liable for money damages to an employer for breach of contract.

The employment contract should specify the length of the contract period; hours the nurse is to work; salary; vacation; sick leave pay; medical, maternal, disability, and liability insurance coverage; educational benefits; and any other benefits or working conditions that the nurse and employer agree on. The employment contract can be terminated legally, without a breach, by completion of all obligations under the terms of the contract or by consent of all parties to the termination.

Respondeat Superior

Under the rule of *respondeat superior*, often called the *master-servant rule*, the master or employer is held liable for wrongful acts of his servant or employee that are done while the employee is within the scope of his employment. The act is usually within the scope of employment if it is the kind the employee is hired to perform, it occurs substantially at the time and place authorized by the employer, and is motivated, at least partly, by the employee's purpose of serving the employer. Although a hospital or other employer may be held liable for the tortious acts of a nurse employee under this doctrine, the nurse is also personally liable for any acts of a tortious nature.

A private duty nurse who is hired and paid by the patient is called an *independent contractor*. The rule of *respondeat superior* does not apply to independent contractors because there is no employer to exercise control over an employee's actions. The patient is the employer of the private duty nurse, and the nurse *alone* is liable for any tortious acts. However, placement services have also been held liable for failure to properly screen health care personnel.

Insurance

The malpractice "crisis" of the 1980s has seen an increasing number of lawsuits in which nurses are named individually along with physicians and hospitals. The public is demanding more accountability from health care providers, and the nurse is perceived as an important member of the health care team, not just an "angel of mercy." The nurse's livelihood should be protected with professional liability insurance to cover the substantial expense of defending a lawsuit. In some instances such insurance may be provided by the employer. The nurse should read the policy and make certain that it covers the nurse's liability as well as the hospital's. If the nurse's liability is not covered, individual insurance protection should be obtained that will (1) pay an attorney to defend a lawsuit filed against the nurse for a wrong alleged to have been committed while practicing nursing, (2) pay any money settlement or judgment awarded in such a lawsuit to the extent of the policy limits on coverage, and (3) pay any bond required if the nurse appeals an adverse decision to a higher court.

Two types of professional liability insurance are available to nurses: claims-made policies and occurrence policies. Claims-made policies must be in force at the time the claim or lawsuit is filed in order to protect the nurse against legal action. If an incident happened in 1989, for example, but a lawsuit was not brought against the nurse until 1991, the claims-made policy would offer no protection unless it were still in effect in 1991. Occurrence policies protect the nurse during a given period of time and cover any incidents that may occur within that time, regardless of when the legal action is filed. A nurse who has an occurrence policy in effect for the period 1989 to 1991 is protected against legal action regarding incidents occurring during that period although the lawsuit may not be filed until 1993.

The nurse should read any policy carefully before purchasing it to ascertain if it covers all aspects of professional work. Some policies exclude certain types of lawsuits, such as those for defamation. Other policies exclude coverage for liability arising from performing certain procedures such as x-ray therapy. The amount payable or limits of the policy coverage should also be considered in light of the type of work the nurse performs and the frequency of lawsuits against nurses in the community where the nurse practices.

If a lawsuit is filed against a nurse who has such insurance protection, the nurse should notify the insurance company immediately and cooperate with the insurance representatives during the course of the lawsuit. Failure to do so may jeopardize the nurse's coverage under the terms of the policy.

Labor Laws

The relationship between nurse and employer is also governed by certain federal and state labor laws and regulations.

Labor Management Relations Act. In July 1974 Congress amended the Labor Management Relations Act to include any hospital, health clinic, nursing home, extended care facility, health maintenance organization, or other institution devoted to the sick, infirm, or aged person. Only public or government hospitals are still exempt from this act, which is designed to prescribe the rights of employees and employers in their relationships with each other and to provide for orderly, peaceful procedures that will protect these rights and resolve any disputes.

The amendment compels the employing institution to engage in collective bargaining with any union or bargaining representative the employees, including nurses, choose. The employer cannot interfere with or discriminate against employees who organize or join a union or unionlike association. Collective bargaining can cover such topics as adequate staffing, provision of modern equipment, inclusion of nurses on hospital committees to voice their views about provision of health care, wages and fringe benefits, grievance procedures, staff development programs, and provision of supportive personnel who will free nurses from nonnursing functions.

This law also regulates the activities of unions and their members, both internally and in their relationships with their employers. If either the employer or employees violate the provisions of the statute, the violation can be brought to the National Labor Relations Board for resolution.

Workers' compensation. Workers' compensation laws are state statutes that provide benefits to an employee who is injured or suffers an occupational disease during the course of his employment. However, not all employers are covered in every state. Some states provide that the employer and employee can choose whether or not to participate in the workers' compensation program. If the employer chooses to belong to the program, an injured employee must accept the prescribed benefits and cannot sue the employer for a larger sum, even if the injury was caused by negligence on the employer's part. The employee who is covered under these statutes does not have to prove, however, that the employer was negligent or that the employee was free of contributory negligence in order to receive benefits as long as the injury arose during the scope and course of employment and the employee gave the employer prompt notice of the injury.

The practical nurse should determine whether coverage is extended to nurses of a specific employer in the state in which the nurse practices. Whether such coverage is provided or not, the nurse may need to consider obtaining disability insurance for income protection because workers' compensation benefits are usually allowed for a certain number of weeks or up to a maximum amount, after which the benefits cease even if the disability caused by the injury is permanent.

Civil Rights

The Civil Rights Act of 1964, as amended, and regulations promulgated thereunder prohibit most hospitals from denying equal job opportunities. Hospitals cannot discriminate in employment, including hiring, firing, compensation, terms, conditions, or privileges of employment, on the basis of race, color, religion, sex, pregnancy, or national origin. Complaints may be filed with the Equal Employment Opportunity Commission, which has the authority to investigate and attempt conciliation of allegations of discrimination and, where warranted, file a lawsuit against a discriminating employer. Federal contractors' employees are also protected by the U.S. Department of Labor Office of Federal Contract Compliance Programs.

Discrimination is also prohibited by other federal and state statutes. Various federal statutes prohibit discrimination on the basis of age for those in the 40- to 70-year-old age-group, mandate affirmative action for employment of the handicapped, and prohibit discrimination in wages on the basis of sex.

State statutes are similar and provide other mechanisms for the employee to challenge an alleged discriminatory act or practice. It should be noted that the statutes of both the federal and state governments prohibit retaliation against an employee who files a complaint of discrimination.

Labor Law Protection

The Fair Labor Standards Act found in Title 29 of the United States Code provides minimum wage and overtime wage protection for qualified personnel. Remedies available to an affected employee include back wages and attorney's fees. "Liquidated damages" may also be awarded. These damages equal twice the amount of the back wages owed to the employee.

The Occupational Safety and Health Act also found in Title 29 of the United States Code requires employers to meet certain standards to protect employees from the risk of injury or illness in the work place. Employees are also protected from retaliation from the employer if they choose to place a complaint against the employer with the Occupational Safety and Health Administration (OSHA). The employee is protected from retaliation even if the complaint ultimately is determined to be without merit. Interest by health professionals in OSHA's regulations has greatly increased in recent years because of AIDS.

As a result of the Employee Retirement Income Security Act and the Consolidated Omnibus Reconciliation Act, found in Title 29 of the United States Code and as Public Law 99-272, respectively, employees also enjoy several provisions that protect their insurance and pension benefits. These laws require extensive notice to employees of their benefits and contain provisions that are designed to preserve and protect these benefits.

All states have unemployment compensation laws that provide some income to the former employee if the employee is laid off or is terminated for reasons unrelated to the employee and beyond the employee's control.

◇   ◇   ◇

Examination of the ethical basis for nursing practice and familiarity with the legal standards that society has decided are appropriate to govern nursing practice will enable the nurse to plan and give patient care responsibly and will protect the nurse's own rights.

◆ *Study Helps*

1. Define the code of ethics for the licensed practical nurse. Explain the significance to you as a practical nursing student.
2. What is meant by legal aspects of nursing? What is the purpose of a license to a practical nurse?
3. How do the code of ethics and legal aspects relate?
4. Define nursing practice acts and their purpose.
5. What is a state board of nursing? What are its duties?
6. What qualifications are needed for licensure?
7. What is the procedure for application for licensure?
8. Distinguish between renewal and revocation of license.
9. What is the most common contract in which you may become involved?
10. What is a tort? Explain the difference between negligence and malpractice.
11. What is meant by invasion of privacy?
12. Define the following:
    • Assault and battery
    • Defamation
    • Drug Abuse Prevention and Control Act
    • Labor Management Relations Act
    • Professional liability insurance
13. State the factors that should be considered when a will is drafted or witnessed.
14. What is the significance of the patient's chart in legal action?

Bibliography

American Hospital Association: Patient's bill of rights, Chicago, 1972, the Association.
Aroskar M: Anatomy of an ethical dilemma, Am J Nurs 80(4):658.
Bernzweig EP: Nurse's liability for malpractice, ed 4, 1987, St Louis, The CV Mosby Co.
Creighton H: Law every nurse should know, ed 5, Philadelphia, 1986, WB Saunders Co.
Cushing M: Verbal no-code orders, Am J Nurs 81:1215, 1981.
Davis A and Aroskar M: Ethical dilemmas and nursing practice, ed 2, Norwalk, Conn, 1983, Appleton-Century-Crofts.
42 United States Code Annotated, Sect. 2000 (e).
Hemelt MD and Mackert ME: Dynamics of law in nursing and health care, ed 2, Reston, Virg, 1982, Reston Publishing Co, Inc.
Levine C et al: AIDS: public health and civil liberties, Hastings Cent Rep 16(6):9, 1986.
National Federation of Licensed Practical Nurses: Code for licensed practical/vocational nurses, 1979.
Northrop CE and Kelly ME: Legal issues in nursing, St Louis, 1987, The CV Mosby Co.
See, for example, Article 45 h, V.T.C.S., Texas Natural Death Act; for explanations see *Vodiga: Euthanasia and the right to die—moral, ethical, and legal perspectives,* Chi-Kent L Rev, vol 51, 1974.
See In the Matter of Conroy, 486 A. 2d 1209 (New Jersey, 1985).
Siks W and Blossun B: Ethics in perspective and practice, Dobbs Ferry, N.Y., 1972, Oceana Publications.
Silva MC: Science, ethics, and nursing, Am J Nurs 74:2004-2007, 1974.
29 United States Code Annotated, Sect. 201-217, 651-678, and 1001-1461.
21 United States Code Annotated, Sect. 801 et seq.
US Department of Health, Education, and Welfare (now US Department of Health and Human Services): Report on licensure and related health personnel credentialing, DHEW Publication No HSM 72-11, Washington, DC, US Government Printing Office.
Ybarra v Spangard, 154 P.2d 687 (Calif, 1945).

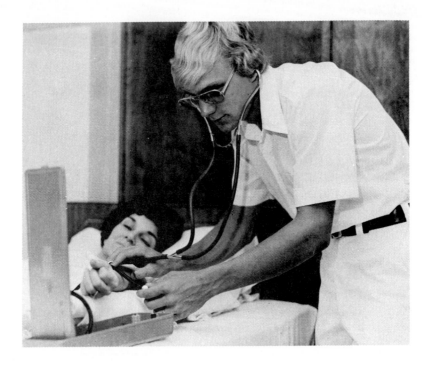

Objectives

At the completion of this chapter the student practical nurse will be able to:

- Discuss the classification system of hospitals.
- Identify members of the nursing team and discuss their roles.
- Elaborate on at least five nursing models.
- List and define the components of the nursing process.

Health Care Facilities and the Patient Care Team

◆ Hospitals

Purpose

Hospitals today have multiple functions. Most people's first thought of a hospital is as an institution designed to meet the needs of the sick and injured. But in the modern hospital there has been an expansion of medical knowledge, technical equipment, and research. The modern hospital provides facilities for the education of physicians, nurses, technicians, social workers, dietitians, therapists, and other health care personnel. It has clinical and research laboratories and takes part in the prevention of disease and the promotion of health through out-patient clinics in the hospital and in outlying community clinics.

The number of hospitals has steadily grown, and they are now a big business, ranking third within the nation's top 10 industries. Approximately 5 million workers, including more than 1.5 million nurses, are employed in hospitals.

Classification

A hospital is classified according to ownership, type of service rendered, length of patient stay, and size.

Ownership may be governmental or private. Government hospitals are operated and owned by federal, state, county or city divisions. Such hospitals include those operated by the Veterans Administration, the Bureau of Indian Affairs, and the United States Public Health Service.

Privately owned hospitals are those owned and operated by labor unions, churches, business or industrial corporations, partners, or individuals. Many hospitals are nonprofit organizations. Hospitals established to ensure profit are called *proprietary* hospitals.

Governmental and private institutions are further classified by service, for example, psychiatric, geriatric, general, and other special fields of medicine. They are subclassified according to the number of beds available: fewer than 25 beds, 25 to 49, 50 to 99, 100 to 199, 200 to 299, 300 to 399, 400 to 499, and 500 beds or more. Federal-operated and state-operated hospitals frequently have the highest bed capacities, totaling 500 or more beds. The largest number of non-profit hospitals fall into the 100- to 199-bed category; city and county hospitals are usually in the 50- to 99-bed category.

When hospitals are classified according to length of stay, they are divided into short term (less than 30 days), long term (30 days or longer), or a combination of both. Short-term institutions far outnumber long-term institutions. Hospitals are using community health facilities to decrease the number of hospital days and the financial cost to patients, institutions, and taxpayers.

As a result of increasing demands for hospital enlargement and remodeling, federal funds are available to individual hospitals under certain conditions. The Civil Rights Act, passed January 3, 1965, assures citizens that hospitals receiving federal funds will not be operated on a segregated or discriminatory basis with regard to race, creed, color, or national origin. It is the primary function of the United States Public Health Service to ensure hospital compliance with signed statements of operation.

The National Health Planning and Resources Development Act of 1974 served as a legal basis for not-for-profit corporations designated and funded by the U.S. Department of Health, Education, and Welfare (U.S. Department of Health and Human Services) as the official health planning and resource development agency for an area. The primary objective of the agency is to provide effective health planning for residents of the health service area. Effective health planning is an activity that identifies health needs and proposes ways to improve the availability, accessibility, and quality of care while being careful to control rising health care costs.

Diagnosis Related Groups (DRGs)

DRGs are the result of the Federal government's attempt to curb health costs. In the past the Federal government reimbursed hospitals for a certain percentage of the cost incurred for caring for Medicare patients. This reimbursement continued for as long as the patients were hospitalized. Now, with the DRG system, the government specifies in advance how much of the hospital bill it will pay for these patients. The amount paid depends on the initial diagnosis, made when the patient is admitted into the hospital. Age, surgery, and complications are considered and can change the allotted period of confinement.

Major diagnostic categories have been established. Each category consists of specific diagnoses, and each diagnosis is assigned a DRG code number. The government has determined the length of hospital stay for a patient in that category. If a hospital can discharge a patient previous to the allotted time, it keeps the profit made from the actual cost of caring for the patient and the amount paid by the government. If the patient stays longer than the allotted time, the hospital suffers a loss. DRGs are expected to save the government millions of dollars in Medicare payments.

Because of continuing changes, such as the DRG system, nurses will need to develop more skills in business and management. Fewer personnel and more acutely ill patients will necessitate utilization of available personnel to their fullest potential. Maintaining a close relationship with the medical records department and maintaining contact with physicians to assure records are complete and accurate will become important and necessary functions for nurses.

Administration

The ultimate governing body of any hospital is known as the *board of directors* or *trustees*. This board defines the philosophy of the institution (for example, to ensure patient care at the lowest possible cost) and its roles and functions, which include patient care, education, research, and community involvement.

The board delegates the administration of the hospital to an administrator or executive director. The administrator or director is responsible for managing the affairs of the hospital, business, and health care. The administrator may or may not have an assistant. In many hospitals there is an administrative council and medical director who function in an assisting or advisory capacity to the administrator or director. The administrative council is composed of designated persons who collectively have the responsibility for all areas in the hospital, nursing and nonnursing. The medical director is responsible for the supervision and practice of the medical staff, interns, and residents. These functions may vary among different institutions.

Department heads govern major areas of operation. Each department head has assistants or supervisors who are responsible for the activities of several areas within a department. A key person is appointed in each specific area to assist the supervisor in carrying out the functions of the department. In the nursing areas this person is called the *head nurse*. The head nurse is directly responsible for patients, nursing care, and personnel in a particular division of the hospital. The head nurse appoints *team leaders*, who assign, guide, and assist team members in the performance of nursing procedures and treatments for the patient. Each has the responsibility for the activities of team members. Team members consist of registered and practical nurses, students, and ancillary personnel. Student practical nurses working as team members render patient care. Their assignments, guidance, and supervision, however, are the responsibility of the practical nurse instructor.

Educational Programs

Educational programs established for medical students, interns, and residents are under the direction of the medical director. In-service educational programs are under the direction of an in-service or educational coordinator. The director of the school of nursing is responsible for the faculty, students, and school curriculum. The faculty consists of instructors, clinical instructors, or a combination of both. The instructor usually teaches basic principles. The clinical instructor implements the application of principles in clinical practice in specific nursing areas. In programs that combine the two, one person functions as both instructor and clinical instructor.

The in-service coordinator or educational director may be responsible to the director of nursing or to one of the administrative council members. The director of the school of nursing is frequently responsible to a member of the administrative council.

Accreditation

Hospital accreditation protects patients and grants recognition to hospitals for services rendered. It stimulates and urges hospitals to conduct ongoing self-evaluation within its structures to initiate continual growth and improvement. Accreditation requires institutions to meet specific standards that include good medical records, quality nursing care, organized medical staff, and adequate clinical facilities.

The accreditation committee consists of representatives from the American College of Physicians, American College of Surgeons, American Medical Association, and American Hospital Association. Surveys are conducted by field representatives, who report their findings to hospital representatives with suggestions for improvement at the termination of the survey and submit a detailed written report to the Board of Commissioners of the Joint Commission on Accreditation of Hospitals. Accreditation provides a means of improving hospital structure, organization, care, and employee morale and ensuring quality care to patients.

◆ The Nursing Team

Hospitals, extended care facilities, welfare agencies, and general health facilities have undergone great changes in education, function, and use of nursing personnel. These changes were necessary to keep pace with new demands in the health field. These new demands include medical and scientific advances, shorter hospital stays, and more complex nursing procedures. Although the supply of nurses is increasing to meet these demands, a shortage of personnel still exists in some areas.

The members of the nursing team included under nursing service today are registered and practical nurses, student nurses, nursing assistants, unit or ward clerks, and, in some hospitals, ward or unit managers. Each of these hospital personnel gives either direct or indirect patient care. Indirect nursing care is performed away from the patient; direct nursing care is performed at the bedside. Through improved educational programs and in-service education programs, the supply of better prepared nursing personnel is constantly increasing.

The Registered Nurse

It is important to know the role of the registered nurse to understand more completely your role as a practical nurse. There are similarities and differences between the two roles.

The registered nurse is a graduate of a college or university nursing program. The program may vary from 18 months to 4 years. The registered nurse has met the legal requirements for registration in the state of practice. This includes successful completion of a written examination, which demonstrates that the nurse possesses necessary technical knowledge and skill. Registered nurses may serve in various positions such as director of nursing service, supervisor, clinician, nurse practitioner, head nurse, staff nurse, or team leader, or they may be employed in private duty, physicians' offices, public health, or industry. Statistics show that the largest number of nurses are employed in hospitals.

The registered nurse assumes the responsibility for patient care in the absence of the physician. This responsibility has been entrusted by the hospital or institution, the attending physician, or both. It is the nurse's duty to know the physical, spiritual, psychological, and social status of each patient. Each nurse is expected to observe and report, as necessary, any significant symptoms or reactions in patients and must see that all prescribed treatments and medications ordered by the physician are given.

As a staff nurse or team leader the registered nurse is directly responsible to the head nurse or, if entrusted with a higher position, the next person in the line of authority. The staff nurse or team leader must teach and supervise fellow team members, make assignments, and coordinate the activities of all personnel in that unit. The patient must be provided quality nursing care through a well-organized, smoothly functioning relationship among team members.

The Practical Nurse

When you finish your program of practical nursing, you will be eligible to write the licensing examination in the state where you are studying or in any state or U.S. territory if you meet the established criteria of that state or territory. Success in passing this examination will give you the title of licensed practical nurse (LPN). This title means that you are a qualified practitioner of nursing, having completed the requirements in an approved program of practical nursing.

A few of the older licensed practical nurses received their licensure by waiver, meaning that they successfully passed the licensure examination even though they did not attend or complete an accredited program in practical nursing. Their past experiences in the field of practical nursing gave them sufficient knowledge to pass the licensure examination. This situation is nonexistent in most states today. Because of the high educational standards currently existing and because of the availability of approved schools of practical nursing, licensure is granted only after the applicant has completed an approved program in practical nursing and has successfully written the state board examination. Because nursing is a scientific and skilled profession, it demands qualified practitioners of nursing to ensure the patient and his family safe and efficient nursing care.

Although programs vary somewhat in different states, the fundamental principles of practical nursing are included in all programs. Plans and ideas are being considered today to establish more uniformity in practical nursing requirements and to establish a universal recognition and acceptance of practical nurses.

You will in all probability be given tasks or functions to perform that require considerable skill and responsibility. An example may be the administration of medications. Remember that certain medications are administered by the licensed practical nurse, but other drugs, more potent and dangerous, are not. Licensed practical nurses are responsible for all their actions. If you assume a position for which you have not been trained, you are liable for your actions. Your particular state legislates laws concerning the functions you may perform as a licensed practical nurse. If you violate these laws, your license can be revoked by the state, and you can be prosecuted.

Statistics show that a majority of recently graduated practical nurses are employed by nursing homes, extended care facilities, home health agencies, and hospitals. By utilizing all members of the health care team to their maximum capacity, these facilities ensure safe, efficient, and effective nursing care for the public.

The Student Nurse

Student nurses may be enrolled in either a registered nursing program or a practical nursing program. Both types of programs must provide good teaching situations. Students of a registered nursing program should be entrusted with responsible positions on the team for both learning and teaching experiences. However, they must be capable of handling this type of situation before it is given to them. They may function first as team members and then as team leaders in clinical settings. In this type of learning experience the registered nurse is often assigned as a team member. In this position the registered nurse is readily available to assist the student in any difficult situations that arise. It gives the student nurse the assurance needed in this new experience, and it safeguards the patient's right to safe, quality nursing care.

As a practical nursing student you should be given situations that require direct nursing care of the patient and include various types of procedures. As a student working under the supervision of the registered nurse or licensed physician, you must learn which observations to make, their significance, and the importance of reporting them to the registered nurse, team leader, or physician. Because you work directly with the patient, you are in a position to observe the patient more closely and to discover his feelings about and reactions to his illness and treatment. With your assistance the registered nurse is more effective, since each team member is depended on to provide information. Your help is needed in caring for the patient. You need adequate supervision to receive instructions, interpret orders, and learn to perform procedures correctly. In this manner you can give competent bedside care without causing harm or distress to either your patient or yourself.

The Nursing Assistant

Nursing assistants are assigned to provide simple nursing care and to perform uncomplicated nursing procedures. They are assigned to either male or female patients.

Nursing assistants give direct care to less seriously ill patients and assist practical nurses and registered nurses in rendering care to critically ill patients. They are prepared for their positions through in-service classes and on-the-job training. Some hospitals have a 2- to 6-week nursing assistant program. Each assistant must attend this program and successfully pass an examination before being permitted to work in the clinical area as a team member.

These employees are taught fundamental principles and procedures such as bedmaking; bathing a patient; ambulation; afternoon and evening care; taking blood pressure, temperature, pulse, and respiration; and the method of distributing fresh drinking water. Formerly, many cleaning duties such as washing beds and units after the patient's discharge and cleaning closets and utility rooms were assigned to the nursing assistant. Today in most hospitals the housekeeping department has taken over these duties. This frees nursing assistants to spend more time with the patient and to render additional nursing care.

The Unit or Ward Clerk

The unit or ward clerk is usually considered one of the clerical nursing personnel. This employee has clerical, administrative, hostess, and public relations duties to perform, as well as much of the paper and desk work. The unit or ward clerk keeps the nursing station area in good order and appearance and coordinates communications for both the registered nurse and team members. The unit clerk is prepared to free the nurse from time-consuming paper work by ordering supplies, making out necessary requisitions, processing physicians' orders, and taking and answering telephone messages other than those involving physicians' orders.

It is helpful if the unit clerk has some secretarial experience and on-the-job training to be more organized and systematic in fulfilling the duties of the job of unit clerk. The unit or ward clerk is frequently responsible to the head nurse. However, if a unit manager is used in the hospital, the ward clerk may be responsible to the unit manager.

The Unit Manager

The position of unit manager is being used in some hospitals; the responsibilities are administrative and are planned to free the nursing personnel for patient care.

The unit manager contacts other hospital departments such as the housekeeping, pharmacy, and dietary departments; is responsible for most of the nonnursing duties on the unit; and answers to the unit coordinator, who is directly accountable to the administrator or administrative assistant.

◆ Nursing Care Models

The interest of every hospital is to render quality, efficient, and economical nursing care. The nursing care model will depend on the hospital and the use of the personnel previously discussed. Nursing care models are created as a result of patients' needs, and they should be given much consideration. There are three general methods of assignment: the functional patient care method, the comprehensive patient care method, and the progressive patient care method.

Functional Patient Care

The functional patient care method is one in which personnel are assigned specific duties such as giving baths, performing treatments, dispensing medications, and starting intravenous fluids. This is the oldest acceptable method of giving nursing care; however, it is not necessarily the best method. With this method the registered nurse has certain duties such as checking physicians' orders; the practical nurse gives treatments; and the nursing assistant gives baths and makes beds. Only a cross section of ward activities is seen in this type of assignment method, and patient care is sporadic and often unorganized.

Comprehensive, Primary Care, and Team Nursing

Comprehensive nursing. In the comprehensive method the nurse has the complete care of all patients assigned for a given shift. This method includes actual bedside care, spiritual and mental needs, and teaching the patient to cope with his condition in the hospital and when he goes home. With this method the nurse has an opportunity to know the patient as completely as possible. Therefore in comprehensive patient care the patient is considered a complete individual, and all aspects of his care are administered by the same nurse.

Primary nursing. Primary nursing is similar to comprehensive nursing, where one nurse is assigned to each patient. The difference between the two is in the length of time the nurse is responsible for the patient's care.

The primary nurse is a registered nurse and is the principal nurse for the patient. She is responsible for planning the 24-hour nursing care of several patients from the day they are admitted to the hospital to the day they are discharged. The primary nurse assesses the needs of the patient and together with the patient and other health personnel formulates a nursing care plan. The primary nurse should be able to demonstrate advanced knowledge and skill. These are generally attained through work experience and continuing education. The primary nurse must have authority, accountability, and autonomy in patient care, and her clinical nursing practice should set an example for other members of the health team.

The associate nurse may be a registered nurse or a licensed practical nurse who has been approved by the head nurse and who has the knowledge and skill to provide direct and total patient care. The associate nurse must be able to follow a nursing care plan, identify the changes that may occur in a patient's condition to alter the planned interventions, and correctly document patient responses. The associate nurse serves as the right hand of the primary nurse, and together they work to provide total holistic care to the patients on their unit.

Team nursing. The team method of assignment is probably the most widely used method today. It provides for the maximum use of all employees' abilities for an assigned group of patients. Team members have total responsibility for these patients. The team may be under the direction of a registered nurse, a licensed practical nurse, or a student nurse from a registered nursing program. The team consists of the team leader, or director, and team members. These members include a registered nurse or nurses, licensed practical nurses, student nurses, and nursing assistants.

The purpose of team nursing is to render quality nursing care to a specified group of patients by using each member of the team to the fullest capacity. The team leader is familiar with all the patients assigned to the team and their disease processes, knows the team members and their capabilities, and plans assignments with this knowledge in mind. The team leader may incorporate both the functional and comprehensive methods of nursing care.

Depending on the type of personnel and their training, the team leader may use the comprehensive method, assigning each team member the total care of particular patients. This service includes medications, treatments, and nursing care. This method may not be advisable to use when the team consists of nursing assistants because they do not have the proper training to perform some of these functions.

The functional method, in a modified form, is often the most commonly used method. The team leader or one of the registered nurses will be assigned to administer the medications to all patients assigned to the team. Treatment and nursing care are given by individual team members for all assigned patients. The team leader or registered nurse may be required to perform advanced or difficult procedures or at least supervise or assist in their performance.

A description of the daily routine of a hospital shift (7 AM to 3:30 PM) using the team method may be as follows:

The team leader receives the report on all patients from the night nurse at 7 AM.

The team leader then adjusts the assignments for personnel. It is advisable to make these assignments the evening or day before.

The team leader checks all patients briefly.

While the leader is performing these activities, the team members are preparing patients for breakfast and serving them their trays.

At 8 AM the team leader gives assignments to team members, including reports on all patients assigned to them.

Team members render the designated nursing care and perform treatments as ordered. They seek assistance if and when necessary.

The team leader administers medications and assists with treatments as necessary.

The team members give feedback of any pertinent information to the team leader.

After morning care has been completed and lunch trays have been served, the leader has a conference with the team members. The conference can be centered around one patient, or it can be a brief report on all or selected patients. It should indicate the patient's needs and possible suggestions made by the group for planning the care of the patient, which are recorded on the written nursing care plans.

This conference is necessary. It helps the team members to realize their importance on the team. It stimulates their interest and encourages them to give better care. It gives them a clearer understanding of their patient as a total individual. It helps the team leader to plan the patient's care. It assists the team leader in knowing the patient and his needs more thoroughly and in discovering significant factors relating to his treatment and care. It helps to gain the understanding, confidence, and support of all team members.

After treatments have been completed, the patients made comfortable, and rooms put in proper order, members can make a final check on the medical record to ensure that nothing has been forgotten or omitted.

At 3 PM the team leader will give a report on all patients to the oncoming registered nurse.

The team method requires the total effort and active participation of all its members.

Progressive Patient Care

Progressive patient care is a concept in which medical and nursing care is carried out according to the degree of illness and the patient's needs, instead of according to cost, sex, and diagnosis. Depending on the hospital, these needs will be broken down into five units, or divisions. Each unit is designed to meet the needs of the individual patient.

Intensive care unit. The intensive care unit is designed to care for critically ill patients. Their conditions may be the result of injuries, surgery, or disease. These patients receive specialized nursing care by trained staff. Often in this area the team method of assignment is used. These units have necessary drugs and lifesaving equipment readily available. A nurse with maturity, good health, emotional stability, and ability to work well under pressure is an asset to this division. A patient is transferred from the intensive care area by written or verbal orders of the attending physician when he believes that the patient no longer requires this type of nursing care.

Intermediate care unit. The intermediate care unit is designed for patients who need a moderate amount of nursing care. Some of these patients are able to help plan and carry out part of their care, such as taking their own baths, being up and about or at least walking to the bathroom, and taking care of their own personal needs.

The procedures performed by health care personnel are of a more routine nature. The functional assignment method may be effective in this area. However, many hospitals today are using the team method.

Teaching in this area is of utmost importance to prepare the patient adequately for the self-care unit. The emotional and physical reactions to illness must be understood by the nurse on this unit to prepare the patient for the future.

Combination of intensive care and intermediate care units. Some hospitals are now combining the two types of care to ensure a continuity of medical care and provide a complete learning situation for the medical personnel receiving training.

Self-care unit. The self-care unit consists of patients who can take care of their own personal needs but still require rehabilitation and teaching. These may be patients admitted for diagnosis, or they may be convalescents. A home-like atmosphere is provided. The patients may have visitors at any time, and they may wear street clothes. They may go to the x-ray or physical therapy department alone, if this is the policy of the hospital. In some hospitals they eat their meals in the hospital cafeteria.

As a nurse on this unit you will have a great deal of time to spend with your patients. You can teach them the use of equipment that they will need to use at home. You can help them to adjust to their illnesses and to adequately care for themselves in their homes. You may need to assist them in adjusting to hospital routines, should they require definite surgery in the near future.

Long-term care unit. The long-term care unit may also be known as the extended care unit. The patients on this unit require nursing care over an extended period of time. The functional or team method of nursing care may be used in this area.

The care of these patients may require the use of more nonprofessional personnel, supervised by the registered nurse, rather than professional help. Teaching and rehabilitation are important for the patient's satisfactory return home. Recreational and occupational therapy are stressed in this unit.

Other Types of Nursing Care

Community health nursing. Community health centers are established in an effort to bring health care into the communities. They are designed to motivate the poor and deprived to seek care freely. Community health nurses can provide many types of patient care in such centers.

Some types of health care provided are (1) prenatal care for maternity patients; (2) psychiatric care such as day care, therapy groups, foster family care, halfway houses, and night care centers; and (3) rehabilitative care, which serves mostly young persons, many of whom are treated for drug addiction. There are also centers for vagrants, where many middle-aged and older persons receive necessary care.

Although the scope and boundaries of these community services vary and still remain issues for continued exploration and improvement, with this type of health care available in the neighborhoods more people will have access to and receive the care they need.

Home health care agencies. The purpose of home health care agencies is to provide home care services essential for maintaining persons at home in the presence of illness and/or disability. Services are directed toward preservation and restoration of health, prevention of disease and disability, and therapeutic care and rehabilitation on an intermittent basis in an individual's place of residence. The service is accomplished by using the services of licensed registered nurses, licensed practical nurses, social workers, dietitians, home health aides, physical therapists, occupational therapists, speech therapists, and other appropriate personnel.

Hospice unit and care. Hospices arose as a reaction to the tried way of caring for the terminally ill patient. The hospice idea tries to overcome the inhumane approach by portraying death and dying as inevitable and normal. To be admitted to a hospice usually requires that a patient have 6 months or less to live. Control over the patient's illness, care, and environment are maintained. Within the hospice unit patients and their families are looked on as one complete unit requiring care. Nurses are able to establish a close relationship with the patient and the family. This allays many of the patient's fears, assists him to die with dignity, and comforts the family members in their time of bereavement.

Private duty nursing. The private duty nurse takes care of each patient on an individual basis. This care may be in an institution, a home, or wherever the patient desires. It may include traveling with the patient. The nurse is paid by the patient or his family and is directly responsible to the patient's physician. If the patient is in an institution, the nurse will be responsible also to the nursing administration.

Group nursing. With group nursing three or four patients share the same nurse. They share the cost and the nursing care rendered. Here the nurse is responsible for the total care of each patient and is paid directly by the patients or their families. It is similar to private duty nursing except the nurse in this situation ministers to three or four patients instead of to only one.

◆ Tools of Nursing Care

Quality nursing care is the goal of every hospital. Its achievement requires using personnel to their fullest potential and planning and evaluating nursing care.

The admission assessment notes (Fig. 1), the nursing care plan and Kardex (Fig. 2), and the discharge summary (Fig. 3) are three useful tools, when used correctly, to assist you in meeting your patient's needs.

The nursing care plan is a decision-making process. It is a problem-solving technique and when applied to a nursing situation is frequently referred to as the *nursing process*. The nursing process is the systematic, intelligent course of meeting patient problems. It describes the thoughts and behaviors of the nurses administering care to patients. It is a design for organizing nursing activity, a means to an end, and a process for understanding and promoting health.

The nursing process involves two people, the nurse and the patient. It is a dynamic communication process, and because of this process behaviors may be affected. For example, the behavior of the nurse may affect the patient, the behavior of the patient may affect the nurse, and the environment may affect both. The interaction process differs with each patient because each patient is an individual and with each nurse because of previous learning, experiences, values, and expectations.

The components of the nursing process are as follows:

1. *Assessment*—the collection of information about the patient obtained from the nursing history, frequent patient observations, physical assessment, the nursing report, and the patient's medical record. With this knowledge base the nurse identifies problems the patient may be experiencing. Assessment is the continuous process by which nurses analyze what they feel, see, hear, and smell, and what the patient verbalizes. There are three general categories of patient problems:
   a. Actual problems that can be observed and noted during the assessment
   b. Potential problems that the patient, because of the disease condition, has a high risk of developing
   c. Possible problems that require additional information before they can be considered pertinent to the patient or ruled out as not relevant to the patient
2. *Planning*—developing the specific plan or method of care that involves realistic goal setting for the patient. Nursing approaches are planned to address the specific problems of the patient that have been identified according to priority of need. The nurse sets short-term goals for the patient's progress after determining the potential that exists for correcting the problems. The established level of recovery for the patient must be realistic. Short-term goals, or

```
                         ADMISSION-ASSESSMENT NOTES

1.  Admission (filled out by admitting personnel)
    Date_____Time_____Previous admissions: No_____Yes_____Date_____
    Age_____Religious preference_____Mode of arrival_____
    T___P___R___BP___Wt___Ht____Urine specimen_____
    Personal belongings and valuables:
    Artificial devices: Hearing aid____Wig____Glasses____Contact lenses_____
    Limbs_____Dentures: Upper_____Lower_____
    Other_____
    Valuables: List_____
    To business office: Yes____No____Receipt_____
    List valuables sent home_____
    Oriented to room: Yes____No_____Side rails explained: Yes____No____
    Do you want a: TV: Yes____No_____Newspaper: Yes____No____
    Visiting hours explained: Yes____No_____
    Physician notified:_____

                                   Admitted by_____


2.  Nursing assessment (filled out by team leader)

    PHYSICAL STATUS:
    Present illness_____

    Symptoms_____

    Past illnesses_____

    Current medications/treatments_____

    Brought medications to hospital: Yes____No____Sent home_____
    Allergies (meds., food, and environmental)_____

    Skin condition or marks_____
    Loss/impaired motion or senses_____
    Habits:
       Diet and eating habits_____
       Bowel habits_____
       Bladder habits_____
       Sleep habits_____

    PERSONAL PROFILE:
    Family structure_____

    Living facilities_____
    Occupation/hours of work_____
    Recreational activities/pastimes_____
    Emotional status_____

    Knowledge of present illness_____

    Teaching needs_____

                                   Team leader_____R.N.
```

Fig. 1

NURSING CARE PLAN				
	Nursing diagnosis	Intervention	Goal	Evaluation
Age	S M D W	Religion	Profession Adm. date	
Standing	Medications	Date	Treatments	Diagnostic tests
PRN				
Room	Name		Diagnosis Doctor	

Fig. 2

expected outcomes, are determined for each identified problem. Long-term goals are established in the form of discharge criteria or the progress of the patient in terms of the expected outcome of the disease and activities at the time of discharge.

3. *Implementation* (intervention)—the initiation and carrying out of the plan that has been established. This means adhering to the plan according to the policies and procedures of the hospital in performing all nursing actions.

4. *Evaluation*—judging the effectiveness of the nursing approaches through examining the patient's responses to the care given. The plan must be revised if the desired effects are not being produced. Evaluation is a continuous process by which the nurse judges the effectiveness of each approach and adapts a plan of care to the patient's responses.

The components of the nursing process may at times be labeled differently, but they are always present. The nursing process, regardless of labels, promotes a systematized, organized way of thinking. The nursing process guides the nurse in decision making, communication, and problem solving. It is a means to standardized care.

◆ Quality Assurance

Quality assurance is a process assuring that quality care is being delivered. It is a formal mechanism used to detect and correct factors that hinder the provision of optimal health care. The methods used to assure quality care must be achievable. Examples of these methods are audits, monitoring, in-service education, performance appraisals, and problem-solving approaches. Quality Assurance is an "umbrella" standard that encompasses all requirements for review and evaluation. Members of a Quality Assurance committee usually are physicians, administrators, and department supervisors.

The *nursing audit* is an evaluation of the quality of care given and is performed by the nursing audit committee. This committee examines and adopts criteria for quality nursing care. The nurse's performance is measured against these established criteria to ensure safe and professional standards of care. Improvement in quality of nursing care will be made on the basis of the audit findings. There may be a need to improve knowledge or performance and in some instances both.

The nursing audit looks at execution of physicians' orders, reporting and recording, application of nursing procedures, techniques, and patient teaching. Outcomes are interpreted in terms of the health-wellness state of a patient after receiving care. The methods for appraising outcomes vary within and among institutions.

The concurrent nursing audit may be carried out several days before discharge. It facilitates prevention of problems, especially for the patient whose care is audited, and is helpful in the evaluation of day-to-day management of care.

◇   ◇   ◇

Although there are various tools and types of methods designed to care for patients, the purpose is the same: efficient, safe, and economical nursing care to every patient. This type of care meets the needs of the patients and promotes satisfaction in the giver and the receiver.

PATIENT DISCHARGE SUMMARY

PATIENT LABEL HERE

I.   HEALTH TEACHING GIVEN WHILE IN HEALTH CENTER: (BEGIN ON ADMISSION)

Regarding:	Instructions Given	Patient	Family	Sign.Other	Verbalized Understand	Return Demonstr.	Given By
☐ ACTIVITY:							
☐ WOUND AND/OR DRESSING CARE:							
☐ DIET:							
☐ MEDICATIONS:							
☐ IRRIGATIONS:							
☐ OTHER (Specify) P.T.-R.T., ETC.							

II. General Condition   Explain
☐ AFEBRILE
☐ PAIN FREE
☐ PAIN CONTROLLED
☐ APPETITE
☐ ELIMINATION
☐ OTHER

SIGNATURE

_____ RN/LPN

PO827   DATE: _____

Fig. 3

III.   METHOD OF DISCHARGE:

☐ RELEASE SIGNED
☐ AMA WITH RELEASE SIGNED BY PATIENT
☐ AMA WITHOUT RELEASE SIGNED BY PATIENT
☐ ELOPEMENT   DATE _____ TIME _____
☐ DR. NOTIFIED DATE _____ TIME _____

DATE OF DISCHARGE _____
TIME OF DISCHARGE _____ | _____ AM _____ PM
☐ EXPIRATION DATE _____ TIME _____ AM _____ PM
POST ☐ YES   ☐ NO
☐ CORONER'S CASE   TIME NOTIFIED_____ AM _____ PM
☐ FUNERAL HOME RELEASE SIGNED
☐ DONATION OF ORGAN (Specify) _____
☐ DONATION OF BODY TO MEDICAL SCHOOL (Specify)_____
MEDICAL SCHOOL NOTIFIED   ☐ YES   ☐ NO

IV.   MODE OF DISCHARGE:

☐ AMBULATORY ☐ STRETCHER   ☐ WHEELCHAIR ☐ WALKER   ☐ CANE   ☐ CRUTCHES   ☐ OTHER _____
☐ PERSON WHO CAME FOR PATIENT AT DISCHARGE: RELATIONSHIP _____
☐ STAFF MEMBER WHO ACCOMPANIED PATIENT TO EXIT AT DISCHARGE _____

V.   ACTIVITIES OF DAILY LIVING AFTER DISCHARGE:

☐ SELF-CARE   ☐ ASSIST   ☐ TOTAL CARE   ☐ PERSON TO ASSIST PATIENT AFTER DISCHARGE _____
☐ WILL NEED ASSISTANCE WITH: ☐ EATING   ☐ DRESSING ☐ ELIMINATION   ☐ MOBILITY ☐ MEDICATIONS   ☐ TREATMENTS
☐ EXPLAIN: _____

VI.   REFERRALS:

☐ NO
☐ YES   WHERE? _____ ADDRESS _____
BY WHOM? ☐ SOCIAL SERVICE ☐ R.N. ☐ M.D.
☐ OTHER _____
☐ TRANSFER FORM COMPLETED AND SENT
☐ OTHER _____

VII.   DISCHARGE TO:

☐ HOME
☐ NURSING HOME _____
☐ OTHER _____
☐ IF OB PATIENT, HOME WITH BABY
☐ IF OB PATIENT, HOME WITHOUT BABY
☐ BABY TRANSFERRED TO _____
☐ HOME HEALTH CARE

VIII.   FOLLOW-UP CARE:

☐ CLINIC APPOINTMENT   ☐ M.D. OFFICE VISIT
☐ OUT-PATIENT TREATMENT ☐ OTHER _____

IX.   SOCIAL SERVICE COMMENTS (IF APPLICABLE)

X.   VALUABLES:

☐ SENT HOME ON ADMISSION
☐ RETURNED TO PT. OR FAMILY AT DISCHARGE
☐ OTHER _____

XI.   PATIENT'S DISCHARGE:

☐ DISCHARGE PRESCRIPTIONS GIVEN TO PATIENT   ☐ INSTRUCTIONS GIVEN TO CONTINUE PREVIOUS MEDICATIONS
☐ NOT APPLICABLE   ☐ OTHER _____

XII.   HEALTH STATUS ON DISCHARGE:

A. Impairments	Comments	B. Mental / Emotional Status	Comments
☐ NONE		☐ ALERT	
☐ SPEECH		☐ ORIENTED	
☐ HEARING		☐ CONFUSED	
☐ VISION		☐ LETHARGIC	
☐ SENSATION		☐ COMATOSE	
☐ AMPUTATION		☐ OTHER	
☐ PARALYSIS		C. Condition of Skin	Description / Location / Comments
☐ CONTRACTURES		☐ GOOD	
☐ FOOT DROP		☐ BRUISES	
☐ OTHER		☐ RASH	
		☐ REDDENED AREAS	
		☐ DECUBITUS	
		☐ INCISION HEALING	
		☐ DRAINING WOUND	
		☐ OTHER	

Fig. 3 (cont'd)

◆ *Study Helps*

1. Why must nursing care undergo changes?
2. Which personnel are included in nursing service today?
3. State and explain the role and functions of the registered nurse.
4. List the two types of student nurses and briefly state their functions.
5. How is licensure obtained?
6. What does the title LPN mean? What is the responsibility of the LPN?
7. Which types of assignments are given to nursing assistants?
8. State the differences between ward or unit clerks and unit managers.
9. How are nursing care assignments made?
10. What does functional patient care mean?
11. What is team nursing and how does it function?
12. What does progressive patient care involve?
13. Explain how the private duty nurse and the group nurse differ.
14. What is included in a nursing care plan?
15. What is included in a nursing assessment?
16. List three community health services.
17. What is primary nursing care?
18. List the four components of the nursing process.
19. What is a nursing audit?
20. What is the duty of the nursing audit committee?

Bibliography

Atkinson LD and Murray ME: Understanding the nursing process, ed 2, New York, 1983, Macmillan Co.
Fromer MJ: Ethical issues in sexuality and reproduction, ed 1, St Louis, 1983, The CV Mosby Co.
Milliken ME and Campbell G: Essential competencies for patient care, ed 1, St Louis, 1984, The CV Mosby Co.
Narrow B and Buschle K: Fundamentals of nursing practice, ed 1, New York, 1982, John Wiley & Sons, Inc.
Rambo BJ: Nursing skills for clinical practice, ed 3, Philadelphia, 1984, WB Saunders Co.

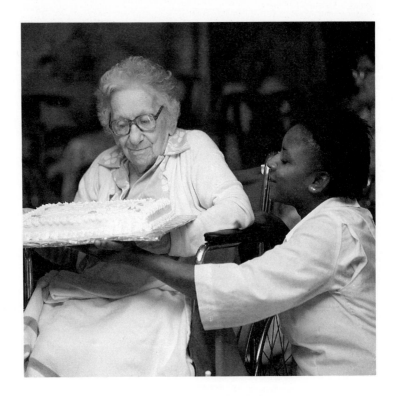

Objectives

At the completion of this chapter the student practical nurse
will be able to:

◆ Describe the five stages of dying.

◆ Describe your role as a nurse in dealing with the patient's visitors
and family.

◆ Identify specific needs of abortion, child abuse, elderly, mentally
ill, and suit-prone patients.

Dealing With Patients Who Have Special Needs

As a student practical nurse and later as a licensed practical nurse, you will be confronted with various types of patient needs. The manner in which you handle these needs will be determined by your understanding of the need, the patients involved, the type of training you have received, and your own personal makeup. Your reactions to situations may vary from those of others. The level of maturity that you have acquired will be an important factor determining your reactions. However, a clear knowledge and understanding of common needs will be an asset to you when confronted with them. A few of the common needs will be discussed in this chapter.

◆ Death

Death is a biological process that culminates at the end of life. When death occurs, all vital body functions cease. A human is born, lives a designated life-span, and dies as the result of the termination of this life-span. This is true of every living organism. The exact length of the human life-span is unknown to anyone. Certain factors play an important role in its termination. Some of these are disease conditions, mental disturbances, accidents, and old age. By the laws of nature every human must die. However, few people are prepared or ready to die. Death is often very difficult to accept, both for the patient who is facing death and for the family who must suffer separation from their loved one.

Every individual develops a concept of death. To a young child death is like sleep. It has no finality. He does not associate death with himself. He does not regard it as something that happens to everyone. Children by 9 or 10 years of age regard death as inevitable. To them everyone lives and then dies. The adolescent regards death as a mystery and ponders an afterlife, and as a teenager he associates death with romance and self-sacrifice. The young adult loves life. He thinks of death as the termination of all things and may display hostile feelings toward it. The middle-aged person is very aware of death. In this age group illnesses may place emphasis on the possibility of dying. The older person often discusses death with his clergyman. He appears to be the most prepared to face death; however, there are stages that all patients pass through before accepting death. These stages are denial, anger, bargaining, depression, and acceptance.

Denial is the stage in which the patient refuses to believe he is going to die. This is a temporary defense that exists in all persons at some time.

Anger is directed at everyone and everything. It is difficult for the nursing staff to manage because it may explode in any direction. You should support the patient in his efforts to make day-by-day decisions.

Bargaining means that the patient wants an extension of time so that he may see someone, do one last task, or wait until some event is passed such as a birth. If possible you should rearrange treatments or visiting hours to try to fulfill the expressed needs of the dying person.

Depression is the preparatory grief stage. The dying person is sad and may withdraw from both his family and the staff. At this time his wishes must take precedence over everyone else's.

Acceptance is the prelude to a peaceful death. During this stage the patient may be tired and weak and dozes frequently. However, you should be aware of his loneliness and not abandon him in his dying stage. Some patients never attain acceptance and will fight to the end. You will have to react to their behavior as it occurs and offer emotional support by being present and listening.

To be of assistance to the dying patient, his relatives, and friends, you must be aware of your own feelings toward death and analyze these feelings. Your approach to death must be realistic. Just as everything you use wears out at some time or other, so does the human body. Sometimes because of excessive use or faulty mechanism, the equipment may have a short life-span. Prolonged use or congenital malformation of organs of the body may shorten the life-span. A healthy appearance does not necessarily mean that all body structures are functioning correctly. All structures have a specific purpose. If one becomes defective, the entire body is affected.

It is difficult to understand that the effect of disease on the body often ends in death. The more difficult situations to understand are deaths that occur as a result of mental disturbances and accidents. Suicide is the taking of one's own life; it is usually caused by a highly charged emotional situation or depressed state. The person who takes his own life may not be considered responsible for this act.

Accidents cause many deaths each year. They may result from carelessness or merely from strange causes or circumstances. This type of death is very difficult to accept because it is so sudden, usually involves healthy individuals, many of whom are young, and produces a state of shock in the surviving relatives. Many emotions are elicited by accidental deaths. Unfairness, cruelty, despair, loss, and rebellion are common emotions displayed. Relatives and friends may feel that God has been unjust to them and to their families. They may begin to wonder if there is a God. If there is, then how could He be so cruel as to allow this to happen? They may rebel against Him and against society. They may become embittered. For a time they may feel that life is not worth living if they must live it without their loved one. But life continues, and the bereaved persons must adjust themselves and their lives to meet this present loss. Some may need help adjusting.

Persons who believe in an afterlife often find death easier to accept than those who do not. They regard death as a temporary separation. They think of it as a state of complete happiness and bliss. They feel relieved that the period of suffering is ended for their loved one. Some feel that the loved one's real purpose in life has been accomplished. They regard life as a journey leading to eternal life, which is a permanent resting place, a place in which all their hopes and desires will be fulfilled. Some think of it as heaven, where the deceased person is enjoying the company of God.

Religious training plays an important part in determining a person's particular feelings about and attitude toward death. You should know the religion of the dying patient and his family to be of real assistance to them in their time of need.

Patient's Feelings

Few persons are ever ready to die. The patient often experiences real fear when death is approaching. He is afraid of the unknown. If he does not believe in an afterlife, then life is terminating with real finality. To this patient death means a complete separation forever from friends and relatives. It means the end of everything. This type of patient clings to every last shred of life.

Patients who believe in an eternity also suffer from uncertainty and fear. They may fear the judgment of God. The Catholic patient may fear condemnation to purgatory or hell for all eternity. Those who regard death as a journey often manifest a degree of peace. However, they still fear the uncertainty of the future.

How should you deal with the dying patient? First of all, know his religion and notify his clergyman if so desired or necessary. Remain with the dying patient if possible. No one wants to die alone. Pray with him, if requested or indicated. Let the patient know that you are there. This can be done by holding his hand, stroking his arm or face, or speaking softly to him. Render the necessary nursing care to afford him comfort. Never speak in his presence as though he were already dead or incapable of hearing what you are saying. The last sense to disappear in a dying patient is that of hearing. He often hears more than you think possible in his condition. If the patient knows that those who care for him are with him, this brings tranquility and peace to him. He feels safe as long as his loved ones are with him. Everyone is afraid of the unknown. However, when it is necessary to venture into it, it gives the frightened person courage to know that someone is with him.

Family's Reaction

The family of a dying patient may react in various ways. They can be emotional almost to the point of hysteria. They may be inconsolable at this time. The best response is to get the family involved in some type of activity. Involvement may take the form of notifying other members of the family or making certain arrangements when death becomes inevitable. The physician may order a sedative to calm a relative. If the relatives are causing a disturbance in the dying patient's room or in the corridor, you should take them to an enclosed waiting room or any other private place. Remain with them until they have composed themselves. This type of behavior may be upsetting to the dying patient, as well as to the other patients in the unit.

Some relatives react in a hostile manner. They may blame the physician or the hospital or both for the person's death. They often say things that they ordinarily do not feel and would not say if they were not emotionally upset. This type of behavior can be irritating to hospital personnel. However, the best manner in which to check these feelings of hostility or resentment is to show kindness and understanding.

The most difficult situation with which you may have to cope is the family who does not react at all. They appear relieved over the possibility of the approaching death of their relative. Their relief is for themselves, not for the patient. They may be interested in the monetary possessions that they have planned to inherit. They are often greedy and will stop at nothing to get what they want. Your normal reaction to this type of situation may be disgust and perhaps hatred. You may wonder how anyone could be so cruel or callous. You are inclined to protect the patient from them. In many cases the dying person has long been aware of his relatives' feelings toward him. This awareness may hurt him and make him feel completely alone. Your greatest service is to remain with the patient and show him that you care about him as a person. He needs someone to be kind to him. In all probability, you will have little effect on the relatives. As a professional person you must always show tolerance and kindness. Your conduct will stand as a monument to your profession. It may have a lasting effect on the relatives although it may not be apparent at the time.

Coping With the Situation

Regardless of which reactions the family may portray, there are certain things that must be done. Everything possible must be done to prevent other patients from becoming upset over the death of another patient. This can be accomplished by closing the other patients' doors and especially the door to the room of the dying or dead patient. Working in a quiet, efficient manner can minimize the attention drawn to this area. Upset relatives can be isolated in a closed waiting room.

Relatives may ask many questions after their loved one's death. If you listen and show that you are interested and concerned, this may be really all they want of you. If they talk long enough, they usually solve their own problems and answer their own questions. Try listening rather than answering in situations such as these. The family must come to its own decisions regarding funeral arrangements and burial. They must decide whether they wish a postmortem examination. If they ask your advice concerning an autopsy, you can explain the meaning of an autopsy to them in simple terms. An example may be: "An autopsy is similar to a surgical operation. The abdomen and sometimes the head are opened, and the organs are examined." You may state the advantages of having an autopsy performed. These advantages include determining the real cause of death, perhaps helping another member of the family who may at some future date have similar symptoms, and helping to increase medical knowledge through this careful and educational procedure. Assure the family that if they do desire this examination, the dead patient will not be disfigured in any way. The family should never be forced into this decision. Usually the physician or house physician seeks this permission. Nevertheless, you may be the person from whom the relatives seek advice. Always refer them to their physician for anything other than a simple explanation.

If the family is indecisive and knows no funeral director, you may direct them to the yellow pages of the telephone directory. The choice should be left to them, and you should not influence them in making it. They can note the various locations and select one that is closest or most suitable to them.

Immediately after the patient has been pronounced dead, the family should be left alone with the deceased, if desired. This privacy should be allowed them. These last few minutes are greatly treasured. It also helps them to accept to some degree their loss and gives them the time needed to compose themselves.

While the body is being prepared, the family should be taken to a quiet, private place where they can discuss the necessary arrangements that must be made. In most hospitals the funeral director must be contacted and a release of the body to the undertaker must be signed before the family is permitted to leave.

The personal belongings of the deceased should be carefully packaged. Valuables should be personally given to a close member of the family, and a note should be made to this effect on the patient's chart. If you are uncertain as to which belongings are the patient's, you may ask a member of the family to help you gather the possessions. After all arrangements have been made and the necessary forms signed as required by the hospital, accompany the relatives to the exit.

After the relatives have departed, the body may be taken to the morgue. The chart must be completed. Use the procedure indicated by the hospital in which you are working.

If religion plays an important part in the burial arrangement and the family members have questions as to whom to contact, refer them to the hospital chaplain, their parish priest, or their minister. These clergymen will give them the necessary information they are seeking and will direct them in these matters.

Death is very personal to the bereaved relatives. The kindness and sympathy that you manifest to them will often be remembered for a long time. You should be helpful to them, but they must make their own decisions. You must control your own emotions if you are to be of assistance to the family. They expect you to be the professional person that your vocation demands at all times.

◆ Single Mothers

Single mothers are faced with complex problems. They have the problem of being pregnant, plus the problem of not being accepted by society. In dealing with these patients the best and most helpful attitude to maintain is that single mothers are not "bad girls" but pregnant women. Your attitude should be neither patronizing nor condescending. Single mothers cannot be stereotyped. They may be from wealthy families or poor families. They may be of any race. They may be brilliant or dull, innocent or hardened. Regardless of their backgrounds, single mothers all have real needs. They need to receive proper medical attention for the existing pregnancy and counseling to help them face reality and make the necessary decisions that will arise as a result of their pregnancy.

Where can they receive help? For single mothers who are still in high school or college, the school counseling service can give them the assistance they need. For those not in school many social service organizations offering this type of help run notices in the newspaper. They are also listed in the telephone directory. Not only do these organizations help provide counseling service, they can also help obtain the necessary medical attention that is required and provide means for livelihood, food, and shelter.

Single mothers face many adjustments. Sometimes they are completely rejected by family and friends.

Homes for single mothers usually have work routines, counseling, rest periods, recreation, and infant care classes for those keeping their babies. These women receive prenatal care, including a balanced diet. They are admitted to the hospital for the delivery of their babies. After delivery they are assisted in completing forms for adoption if desired or in making living arrangements and finding employment.

Attitudes are changing regarding single mothers. Many couples who do not believe in traditional marriages are having planned children who are being reared by a single parent. Today more parents are beginning to accept responsibility for a daughter in this situation, allowing her to remain at home during the pregnancy. Single motherhood still presents an emotional situation to which the unmarried mother, family, friends, and society must adjust. Professional counseling can assist the girl and her family.

Professional counseling is offered to the single mother by various agencies. This type of service should never be forced on anyone; it should be a personal choice and decision. The function of such counseling services is to help these mothers establish themselves as individuals, accept themselves as they are, and make plans for the future.

A major decision for the single mother is whether to keep the baby or put it up for adoption. Neither adoption nor keeping the infant should be urged or insisted on. The mother must make the decision; however, she must be given both alternatives so that these may be explored in an unhurried manner.

The woman must adjust to the pregnancy itself. This adjustment involves physical and emotional factors. She may suffer from physical symptoms such as morning sickness or a feeling of distressing fullness. General mood swings will also occur. At the beginning of the pregnancy she may have mixed feelings of elation and depression because of the physiological adjustment of her body to pregnancy. As the pregnancy progresses, the mother may be thrilled and awed with the impending birth of the child she has nourished and helped to form, or she may feel guilt and shame.

The period after delivery may be extremely difficult for the single mother who has decided to have her baby adopted. It is the policy of many organizations to show the baby to the mother one time only. It can create an emotional crisis for the mother to give her baby to someone else. This is the reason that professional counseling is continued after delivery until the mother has made satisfactory adjustment to postpartum life.

The adjustments of the single mother are numerous and difficult; she does not need or desire punishment, lectures, or censure, but rather love, understanding, and hope. She should be treated with respect and dignity and not spoken about in whispered tones that tend to portray her as being "different" from other pregnant women. Be considerate but not patronizing.

◆ Abortion Patients

Since the 1973 decision of the Supreme Court a pregnancy may be terminated at the request of the woman. Interpretations of the decision will vary from state to state and institution to institution.

With liberalization of abortion laws in the United States and abortions being performed legally, you will have to take a close look at your own attitudes and feelings. Abortion patients require understanding, kindness, and psychological support as well as regular nursing care to meet their needs. If you feel you are unable to meet the patient's total needs, discuss this honestly with your instructor, who will help you to cope with the situation in a realistic and mature manner. Employers have a right to know your beliefs regarding abortion and sterilization.

◆ Hostile, Aggressive Patients

In this chapter the hostile, aggressive patient is one whose activities are forward and exceed normal standards as a result of a driving inner force and excessive energy. The activities are willful acts that are contrary to acceptable standards of behavior.

The hostile, aggressive patient can become a real problem on a general nursing division. At first glance it may be difficult to understand the actions of this type of patient. It is easy to forget that sickness sometimes brings with it regression to former stages of development that may vary with the individual patient. A patient's defenses are down when he is ill. He often will express his true self at a time like this. Emotions that have been suppressed will find a release in some form or other.

Often the hostile, aggressive patient has had a strict childhood background. As a child he may have developed fears because of training that was harsh, prematurely instituted, and sometimes exaggerated. This type of control may have extended itself to an inhibition of even normal, healthy activity. Initiative may have been blocked. Spontaneity has often been sacrificed, and continuous defensive efforts must be made to judge authority figures and their wishes. Such a child becomes a "little angel," overly good, essentially timid, and noncontributing. He may have been forced to repress his anger. As a result this repressed hostility has grown until rigid defenses are needed now to control it. When a patient finds himself in a position in which his defenses are weakened, some of this repressed hostility may manifest itself in one or more of these symptoms: severe constipation, diarrhea, sleep disturbances, enuresis, or sexual advances.

The most threatening and difficult situation that may confront the female practical nurse may be advances made by the aggressive male patient. These advances are frightening because the female nurse is unsure of how to cope with them. She regards them as frightening and improper. By all means they are to be discouraged and dealt with adequately. A few suggestions may be helpful for those nurses who are ever confronted with this type of situation.

Always be in control of the situation. Act according to professional decorum. Do not let the patient know that you fear him. Accept the situation as a normal occurrence but one that you will neither tolerate nor accept. If the advances are made verbally, change the subject. If this diversion fails, then state in a quiet but emphatic voice that you do not enjoy this type of conversation. If the patient continues despite your admonition, leave the room as soon as possible and report the incident to the team leader or head nurse.

If the advances are made by physical contact, such as grabbing your hand, trying to kiss you, or attempting to touch certain areas of your body, try to withdraw from the patient. If it is impossible because of the force he is exerting, tell him to stop this type of behavior immediately. Also, tell him that the incident will be reported to the hospital authorities. The patient must be made to realize that this behavior is inappropriate and that you as a professional person will not tolerate it. This may be referred to as *molestation,* which is a violation of a person's rights.

Molestation is the touching of another person's body without consent. A nurse does touch the body of a patient in the performance of duties. However, when a patient signs himself into the hospital, he gives the hospital and those caring for him permission to perform whatever duties are necessary. Therefore the nurse functions under this implied permission of the patient and is not guilty of molestation. The patient does not have any type of permission to touch the body of the nurse, and you as a nurse should not allow this in any form.

In nursing, a belligerent patient differs from an aggressive, hostile patient in that he is combative and may show violence in words or actions. Additional help is usually supplied when rendering care to a patient in this condition. This type of behavior is often demonstrated by the alcoholic or emotionally disturbed patient.

◆ Shy, Withdrawn Patients

The shy, withdrawn patient is one who is quiet and does not express his feelings. This type of person often has a weak personality. He is excessively timid and afraid to mix with others. He may have demanded from his parents or his marriage partner an excessive amount of protection. He usually lacks the moral courage to stand up to a difficult situation. This type of patient tends to accept any illness that may develop and is frequently in a state of mental and physical weakness. He easily accepts defeat and becomes apathetic. He often shows no desire to recover because recovering involves the responsibility of returning to normal life. He avoids anxiety-producing situations. As a patient he must be coaxed, or at least encouraged, to eat, take medicine, or make any attempt to recover adequately. He usually will do what he is told but nothing more. This patient needs understanding, sympathy, and friendly encouragement. This regard will give him a feeling of trust and confidence in you as a nurse and will also give him the incentive to help himself.

If a patient is prone to this type of behavior, hospitalization may exaggerate these symptoms. Hospitalization is a frightening experience to many patients. They feel insecure and are uncertain about the outcome of their illness. They are often afraid to express their feelings because they fear ridicule from their families and the hospital staff. They must be encouraged to express their feelings. If they feel that they can trust you, they will communicate their feelings either in words or in actions. They must be helped to accept their true roles as individual persons and as members of society.

◆ Drug Abuse Patients

Drug abuse, particularly among the young, is a big problem today. Drug abuse is not confined to urban ghetto areas. Affluent suburbia and rural communities are equally troubled. Members of all age groups abuse drugs. Drug use has now spread from college students to high school and junior high school students as "the thing to do."

There are many and varied programs available to the addict. With the increasing awareness of substance abuse as a health problem and less social stigma, more individuals are now seeking help. With this increase in knowledge more programs are available. Prevention programs such as health clinics and schools are available in community health settings. Care units offer inpatient, partial hospitalization, and day and evening outpatient programs. Psychologically the aim is toward control of self.

You must observe drug abuse patients carefully for signs of withdrawal or evidence that drugs are being obtained from inside or outside the hospital. They may attempt to hide pills, especially during the early phase of withdrawal. The addict needs extra support; therefore your role is one of support and nonjudgmental participation.

◆ Alcoholic Patients

Alcoholism is an illness not peculiar to any particular kind of person. It affects people regardless of residence, age, sex, political affiliation, intelligence, social position, color, wealth, or occupation.

Alcohol is the most widely abused drug. In the United States, out of 10 million problem drinkers 6 million are estimated to be alcoholic. At the present male alcoholics outnumber females about 5:1 but this ratio is decreasing. Although men appear to have more drinking problems in their 20s, women most frequently are in their 30s or 40s. Alcoholism also affects the elderly population, perhaps as many as 90%. Although alcoholic treatment programs have been established for men for several years, a growing awareness of the problem in women is reshaping rehabilitation programs to include women's needs. As a student practical nurse you may come in contact with an alcoholic patient of any age and on any of the nursing divisions, including pediatrics.

Some characteristics of an alcoholic patient are denial, impulsiveness, evasion, projection, low frustration tolerance, ambivalence, manipulation, remorse, and low self-esteem. This list is not all inclusive, and not all alcoholics will display all of these characteristics. If you can recognize and accept such behavior as a part of your patient's alcoholism, you can better meet your responsibilities in giving total patient care.

Denial

The alcoholic almost always has difficulty in recognizing drinking or alcoholism as a problem. Although it may be perfectly clear to you, your patient's family, and many other people, your patient may not believe that this is really a problem.

Impulsiveness

The alcoholic often does things on the spur of the moment, without considering the outcome of the actions. The alcoholic is capable of understanding the results of his actions but does not or cannot take the time to consider these actions before he acts, such as when taking the first drink.

Evasion

The alcoholic will hide drinking and will try to avoid any reference to it. The alcoholic will talk about the weather, financial difficulties, or family problems in an effort to stay as far away as possible from discussing the matter of drinking.

Projection

The alcoholic generally attempts to rely heavily on the protective method of blaming his drinking problem on other people or circumstances. The alcoholic sees someone else as being responsible for the difficulty. For example, if the other person would change, then there would be no alcoholic problem.

Low Frustration Tolerance

Little things seem to upset the alcoholic more than they upset other people. The alcoholic seems unusually sensitive to criticism, anger, or other situations that other people would not notice.

Ambivalence

The alcoholic is extremely torn between not drinking and getting another drink. The alcoholic must be given every opportunity to recognize this ambivalence. If you are intolerant of either abstinence or drinking, you deprive the alcoholic of the opportunity to understand himself as completely as possible.

Manipulation

The alcoholic is a master at manipulating people and situations to his own advantage. The alcoholic will frequently get people to make special arrangements for him, vouch for him, protect him, or take some risk for him. After these things have been done for an alcoholic, the alcoholic will frequently start drinking again.

Remorse

The alcoholic experiences a great deal of remorse; sometimes it is so great that the alcoholic can no longer live with it and must have another drink. Increasing the remorse of an alcoholic by shaming, scolding, or belittling can serve only to intensify the problem.

Low self-esteem

Perhaps the most overlooked characteristic of the alcoholic is his low self-esteem. Low self-esteem often goes unrecognized because it is masked by an air of confidence ("I can do anything; I have money, friends, and influence") that is exhibited by the alcoholic. Because he has fooled others for so long, it is difficult for the alcoholic to recognize low self-esteem.

◇　◇　◇

You should be aware of the treatment plan your alcoholic patient's physician has prescribed and reinforce and support both your patient and the family in following this plan, whether it be referral to a rehabilitation center or to Alcoholics Anonymous.

◆ Child Abuse

Child abuse or neglect is a serious and complex behavior problem. In all states, the Virgin Islands, and the District of Columbia, hospitals or other health care providers are now legally responsible for reporting suspected cases of child abuse. Child abuse or neglect should not be ruled out when a child is seen with long bone fractures, burns, bruises, scars, welts, cranial trauma, old fractures, or starvation. Further investigation is warranted in many of these cases.

The details of procedure and substance for reporting abuse or neglect may vary slightly from one state to another. Information needed to investigate child abuse will usually include name, age, address, persons responsible for the care of the child, and the nature and extent of the possible abuse.

As a student practical nurse who observes a child in the emergency room or the pediatric unit and suspects child neglect or abuse, you should immediately notify your instructor.

◆ Suit-Prone Patients

The suit-prone patient is usually a person who is generally unhappy and dissatisfied with all parts of life and therefore is more likely to bring suit for malpractice when something goes wrong than any other type of patient.

Because of the general public's awareness of the legal responsibilities of the physician, nurse, and hospital, lawsuits are brought much more readily for real or imagined negligence. Therefore you must know how to prevent malpractice claims.

Most nursing malpractice suits are caused by the patient's dissatisfaction with care. Using good nursing practice, based on sound knowledge and skill, and acting as a reasonably prudent person under similar circumstances will make you less likely to be involved in a lawsuit. If you assess the individual's total needs, listen to the individual, and explain your actions, the patient will probably accept the care. If you are aware of a suit-prone patient, alert co-workers, keep accurate records, and notify your instructor, who will assist you in dealing with this type of patient.

◆ Elderly Patients

In 1935 the special needs of the elderly became publicly acknowledged with the introduction of Social Security. Retirement was forced on many economically unprepared older persons, leaving them with little hope for the future. As a result many people must live on a fixed income, which does not change as prices rise. This creates needs in areas such as obtaining food, paying utility costs, finding adequate living quarters, and providing coverage for medical care.

Physical changes and the health needs of aging affect all aspects of the older person's life. The frequent feelings of loneliness, indecision, insecurity, helplessness, confusion, and rejection, as well as mental deterioration, must be considered. The physiological changes of aging may include impairment of the senses with maladjustment. The aging person's response and reaction time may be slowed. These changes may make it difficult to solve problems and carry out everyday activities. Whether the source of changes is physical, physiological, or sociological, the whole person responds to the changes.

The field of geriatrics is now considered a specialty. A Division for Geriatric Nursing was included in the 1966 ANA convention. This was important because now nursing recognizes that the elderly have the same health care needs as do people of other age-groups. As a gerontological nurse it is important to assist the older person to identify unmet needs and the resources for meeting these needs. Although personal independence is to be encouraged, as a student nurse you must be aware of the normal changes brought about by the aging process and, using patience, help the patient to maintain dignity by resuming as active a life as possible.

New technologies are being developed that may lessen some needs of the elderly and may greatly increase their level of activity. Some of the technological achievements are better eyesight—with the use of lasers a cataract can be removed in minutes; better hearing—with improved hearing aids and implants; better memory—researchers are discovering new ways to restore memory; and less fear of approaching death—with thanalology (the study of death) people are learning ways to cope with death. Not only curing physical and mental ailments will help the elderly, but also improved television programs will help. Large screens will help those with eyesight loss, subtitles will help those with hearing loss, and remote control will help those who cannot leave their bed or chair. These improvements will bring sports, movies, and current events into the home for the elderly to enjoy.

Some surveys have shown that by the year 2030 the number of Americans 65 years or older is expected to be 64.3 million. The fastest growing group will be those 85 years and older. White women have the longest life expectancy, followed by black women. As our aging population increases we must assume a leadership role in changing society's attitudes about the elderly so they can obtain a higher quality of life.

◆ Elderly Abuse

The elderly are suffering abuses such as neglect, physical assault, threats, and financial losses. Many are left in bed with soiled linens and clothes. They may have bruises which are said to be from falls. The family may threaten them with being placed in a nursing home, so the elderly will usually remain quiet about being abused.

The abuse frequently comes from a son, daughter, or spouse, which may make the elderly ashamed to tell that their own family could do such a thing. It is harder to recognize abuse in the elderly because many are unable to be out in the community where they can be seen. Abuses and neglect may occur in institutions in the form of not keeping the elderly and their surroundings clean, inadequate food, and rough treatment by the workers. The elderly will frequently remain silent because they feel they have no other place to go.

The elderly abuse issue is now starting to be addressed by most state legislatures, universities, and conferences. There are speakers available in some areas on elderly abuse. State laws vary as to the reporting of elderly abuse. Be familiar with the laws of your state.

As a student practical nurse who observes the elderly and suspects neglect or abuse you should report to your instructor, who can advise you what sources are available in your area to help the elderly.

◆ (AIDS) Patients (Acquired Immunodeficiency Syndrome)

AIDS is an illness that is no longer associated with homosexual or bisexual persons, or IV drug users. It is a bloodborne disease and given the right circumstances, AIDS can infect anyone. As one report points out, for every child who meets the Centers for Disease Control (CDC) definition for AIDS, there may be another 2 to 10 infected with Human Immunodeficiency Virus (HIV).

AIDS carries a social stigma. Men, especially, fear being labelled as homosexuals should they develop AIDS. The parents of many AIDS babies do not want them and the babies become wards of the state.

We all have personal views about AIDS. As nurses caring for patients with AIDS, we must examine our own feelings. In some cases the patient's family or friends may also be infected with AIDS. Whatever the situation, it is important to be accepting and caring of the patients and their families and friends regardless of their situation.

If the nurse does not recognize lifestyles that differ from the usual, then it will be difficult to care for the AIDS patient and family.

It is the nurse's responsibility to ensure confidentiality for all patients, including the AIDS patient. Information should be given only to those health care professionals providing care for the individual. Information given to the wrong person about an AIDS patient could cause the patient to lose his job, home, and insurance. Some states have passed legislation to protect the privacy of AIDS patients.

Anger is frequently seen in AIDS patients. It may be directed at themselves for having taken a risk. If they have received a contaminated transfusion or because there is no cure available to them, anger may be directed toward the medical profession. The nurse needs emotional stamina but also needs to have a caring manner when patients, families, or friends are showing their anger.

Because the patient usually dies, care of the AIDS patient is demanding. Nurses who begin to feel depressed, fatigued, or helpless should seek a support group and deal with their feelings openly. Some states are beginning to require AIDS education for nurses before licensure or relicensure to increase their knowledge in this area.

Because there is no cure at the present time, only symptomatic treatment is available for AIDS patients. Nursing care should take into consideration each patient's special needs and implement the care needed to meet them.

◆ Helping the Patient To Accept and Live With His Disease Condition

A patient cannot really accept his disease condition until he knows and understands it. This is his right. Just how much he is to be told and when he is to be told varies with the individual patient, his family, and his physician. The nurse who attempts to fulfill this function needs a good deal of psychological insight and understanding of the patient's personality to determine a wise course of action. It is certainly not desirable for you as a practical nurse to give this type of information. It is your responsibility to relate the patient's anxiety over the matter to your head nurse or team leader. Nevertheless there are some things that you can safely say to the patient. If a patient were to ask you, "Why are they doing this test?" you can safely answer him, sincerely and with concern, "These tests are being carried out so that the physician may find out definitely what is the matter with you." A simple explanation of the test may allay the patient's fears. In unknown situations the patient may be prone to build up imaginary horrors far worse than anything that is likely to happen. Never name the medications or types of dyes used in procedures because patients often tell their friends and relatives the name of a particular medication or tablet and may try to persuade them to take it also. Frequently they may have read an inaccurate report about the medication. As a result they may have distorted ideas about its effect on them and develop a fear of taking it.

It is the responsibility of the physician to determine how much information the patient is to be given. Sometimes the physician explains disease conditions in such a way that the patient is confused. Later the patient may ask the nurse to explain again what the doctor was trying to tell him. The nurse should know what the physician has told the patient before entering into a full explanation of the disease condition. The best way to gain this information is from the physician. In some cases the nurse may ask the patient to explain what he thought the physician was saying. If medical terminology was the stumbling block for the patient, a simple explanation may prove helpful. A rule to follow is "Never explain anything to a patient unless you know what you are trying to explain." Never bluff your way through an explanation. It is unfair to the patient and to your profession. Misinformation can be harmful.

After the patient is informed and understands his disease condition, the nurse can assist the patient in rehabilitation by use of a positive approach. It is easier to accept something positive rather than something negative.

The patient suffering from a crippling disease can many times lead a productive life. With the aid of physical therapy and artificial devices, he may be taught to care for his own needs and pursue various occupations and recreational activities. Before this goal can be achieved, the patient must develop a desire to set such a goal. You can be of assistance to him in this area. Because you work so closely with him, ministering to his different needs, you can often give him the confidence he needs. Your trust in the patient is many times sufficient to create this desire in him.

If the patient is completely helpless and still has full mental capabilities, he can be taught to use his mind rather than his hands or legs. He can further his education and find joy and happiness by reading, watching television, and listening to music. He can remain the head of the house, if this was his former position, by assuming and planning the household activities and finances. This will take a great deal of adjustment, but it can be done.

If he is not mentally alert, the patient may live in his own little world. He is happy because he is not cognizant of his former activities or of the world about him. He may find pleasure in making up fictional stories in which he is the main character. He is oblivious of all around him.

Can there be a positive side to cancer? In some cases the patient will die as the result of the disease process; it may take weeks, months, or even years. Can you be sure that you will not die today or tomorrow? Death is as uncertain for you as for the patient with cancer. He may have many happy days to enjoy with his family. If he can learn to live day by day, he can enjoy much happiness. Many new drugs and radiation therapy have destroyed cancerous cells and slowed their growth.

If the patient's condition is terminal, he needs psychological, physical, and religious support. Encourage him to talk with his clergyman. However, he should not be forced into this. Listen to him. At such times of crisis the patient often looks for a sympathetic, understanding listener. Sometimes you will be the one who can bring him the solace he is seeking. Your understanding may supply him with the courage he will need to face death bravely and peacefully. Death may be the blessing that will end his continuous suffering. By having his physical needs attended to with kindness and empathy, some of his psychological needs for love, affection, and acceptance will be met. Many times it is more difficult to help the family to accept the situation than to help the patient.

◆ Dealing With the Patient's Family and Friends

Relatives and friends are important not only to the patient but also to the nursing staff. The patient is often lonely and longingly waits for his family. The nurse can gain real insight into the patient's needs by talking with relatives and friends. Many emotional, physical, and environmental factors can be discovered through these interactions. The family may help the nurse to decide on the appropriate approach to use for this particular patient.

If you can establish favorable relations with relatives and friends, they are likely to be cooperative and helpful. It is true that the patient's relatives and friends can at times present problems to the nursing staff in its daily routine. Some people exempt themselves from rules and visiting hours. They drop in to see the patient whenever it is convenient for them. They forget that certain functions or duties for the patient's comfort have priority. They may resent being told that they may visit only during the prescribed visiting hours. If you explain in a nonassuming, quiet voice these rules of the hospital and their purpose, often these persons will be more willing to conform to them. If they persist, this should be reported to the head nurse, who will cope with the situation.

When it becomes necessary to perform a procedure during visiting hours, ask the family or friends to kindly wait in the corridor or the waiting room for a few minutes. You may add that this procedure cannot wait until later. If you show them kindness, consideration, and respect, they will be willing to cooperate with anything that is of benefit to the patient. Remember that the patient, his family, and friends are guests in the hospital and should be treated as such.

Because of the crippling or finality of some disease conditions, families sometimes do not readily accept the sickness or misfortune inflicted on one of their loved ones. They tend either to reject it as nonexistent or to rebel against it. This rebellion may be against God, the medical profession, or society. The same procedure that is used to help the patient can be used to help the family. The family must know and thoroughly understand the disease conditions and its implications, effects, and limitations. They must be helped to accept the condition before they can be of assistance to the diseased patient. Arrangements for the family to talk with the physician should be made at your earliest convenience. The help of the social service department may be sought to plan and contact various agencies that render the assistance needed. The family must be given understanding, guidance, and support. However, they must make their own decisions. The patient needs the family's help and is dependent on them. He senses and reacts to their reactions to his illness. Sometimes their clergyman can be of assistance. A positive approach to the patient and his family must be used in order to be effective. All must cooperate in the process of adjustment no matter which type of illness is involved. The degree of adjustment may necessarily differ, but it must be made. Its success depends on the persons involved and their acceptance of the illness.

Bibliography

Barrick B: Caring for AIDS patients, Nurs 88, 18:50-59, Nov 11, 1988.

Edelman C and Mandle CL: Health promotion throughout the life span, St Louis, 1986, The CV Mosby Co.

Estes, NJ: Alcoholism, ed 3, St Louis, 1986, The CV Mosby Co.

Gill J: The development of persons, Hum Develop 2(1):31, 1981.

Gress LD and Bahr SRT: The aging person—a holistic perspective, St Louis, 1984, The CV Mosby Co.

Hamilton PM: Basic pediatric nursing, ed 5, St Louis, 1987, The CV Mosby Co.

Keller MJ: Toward a definition of health, Adv Nurs Sci 43(1):43-52, 1981.

Kinney J and Leaton G: Loosening the grip: a handbook of alcohol information, ed 3, St Louis, 1986, The CV Mosby Co.

Kübler-Ross E: On death and dying, ed 4, New York, 1971, Macmillan, Inc.

Nichols EJ: The influence of cultures and heritage on the aging process. Paper presented at the Regional Forum on Aging, Kansas City, Mo, May 26, 1983.

Wohl PF: Therapeutic relationships with the elderly, J Gerontol Nurs 6(5):260-266, 1980.

◆ *Study Helps*

1. What determines the way you meet the special needs of your patients?
2. What is death?
   • List and explain the five stages of death.
   • State and explain an individual's concept of death as he matures.
   • Why are accidental deaths so difficult to understand?
   • How does religion affect the acceptance of death?
   • What can you do to assist a dying patient?
   • State and explain the family's reaction to death.
   • How can you be of assistance to the family?
3. Which complex needs do the elderly present?
   • What are their needs?
   • Where can they receive help?
   • What should be your attitude toward them?
   • What adjustments must they make?
4. Define and explain what is meant by the term *hostile, aggressive patient.*
   • Explain what is the most threatening and difficult situation for you as a practical nurse.
   • How should you cope with the situation?
   • What is meant by molestation?
   • Explain why the nurse is not guilty of molestation.
   • How does the belligerent patient differ from the hostile, aggressive patient?
5. What are the needs of the AIDS patient?
   • What are his reactions to illness?
   • How can you be of assistance to him?
6. What is the first step in helping a patient or his family to accept his illness?
   • What information can you as a practical nurse give to the patient or his family?
   • Which measures can be used to assist an invalid patient to adjust to his illness?
   • What assistance can you give to the seriously ill patient?
7. Explain the role of relatives and friends in the hospitalization of a patient.
   • How can you gain their cooperation?
   • How can you be of assistance to them in times of stress or crisis?
8. List three changes that take place in an aging person's life.
9. In which year was the abortion law liberalized?
10. What is your responsibility when you suspect child abuse?
11. List three characteristic behaviors that an alcoholic patient may display.

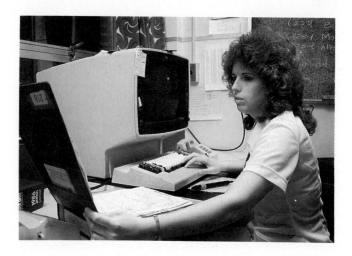

Objectives

At the completion of this chapter the student practical nurse will be able to:

♦ Discuss the purposes of three types of health clinics.

♦ List at least five areas in which the licensed practical nurse may find employment.

♦ Discuss the advantages versus the disadvantages of working in five different areas of employment.

♦ Discuss the licensed practical nurse's role in public relations.

9

Practicing the Vocation

Because public health, industry, and private and general duty nursing absorb many licensed practical nurses, it may help you to discuss these areas in some detail. A clear understanding of each may help you in making your future choice in the specific area that is of interest to you.

◆ The Licensed Practical Nurse in Public Health

Today public health nursing accepts the licensed practical nurse. In this area you may be active in either local or state programs. As a visiting nurse you represent a voluntary community agency. As a public health nurse you represent an official health agency.

Most agencies provide means of transportation, which may be in the form of a car, bus fare, or reimbursement for gasoline and depreciation of your own car. The areas are mapped in such a way that you will not usually have to travel too extensively. This means that you can provide care to more patients in less time. Your work, however, is not limited to rendering care to patients in their homes. It also includes work in school health activities and various types of clinics.

Some of the school health services that are rendered are as follows:
1. Appraising health of faculty and students through
    a. Physical examinations
    b. Dental examinations
    c. Psychological examinations
2. Counseling students, parents, and faculty with regard to health problems
3. Follow-up services in securing correction of remedial defects
4. Assistance in discovery and education of handicapped children
5. Prevention and control of communicable diseases, including immunizations
6. Provision of emergency service in case of injury or sudden illness

Following are some types of clinics:
1. *Maternal and child health clinics*—attempt to improve the hygienic conditions of

maternity, infancy, and childhood and offer prenatal and infant care, including health education
2. *Crippled children clinics*—investigate the prevalence of crippling conditions and provide supplementary aid in rehabilitation of the children affected
3. *Mental health clinics*—help to assess the extent of mental hygiene services needed in a community, carry on educational programs in this area, and offer assistance to affected persons

Other services rendered to the public include prevention, detection, and treatment of communicable and social diseases.

If you are interested in working in the field of public health, the first and most basic qualification that you must possess is the ability to accept and work easily with all types of people. This does not mean doing everything for them but rather teaching them to help themselves.

As a licensed practical nurse you will be supervised by a registered nurse. Your assignment will be made according to your nursing abilities and your personality. You must know or learn the area to which you will be assigned. You must be alert and observant. You must be capable of making accurate decisions in accordance with your position in nursing. The workweek usually consists of an 8-hour day, 5 days a week, with holidays and weekends free. Salaries are comparable to those paid in institutions.

The challenges, variety of people and situations, and ideal working hours entice many licensed practical nurses to enter this field of nursing.

◆ The Licensed Practical Nurse in Occupational Health

Most industrial plants are required to have health programs for their employees. These programs are under the supervision of a physician and a registered nurse, often with a licensed practical nurse working as an assistant. If you choose to work in industry, you must know the duties performed by each level of employee, ranging from the unskilled laborer to top administrator. This information is needed to help plan and carry out necessary accident prevention programs. Because you will be working closely with both employer and employee, you must understand the overall industry and its functions in order to meet both their personal and health needs.

Many industries require preemployment physicals, as well as yearly physicals. For particular reasons some industries may require these physicals more often. Most industries that provide health programs and employ nurses to staff these programs also have an emergency program. You may administer first aid as indicated. You may be required to test vision and hearing. You may be expected to keep health records current on all employees. Your job responsibilities may vary greatly, depending on the industry and its specific type of work.

The hours are usually desirable. In some places you may be asked to rotate shifts. Salaries are higher than those paid in institutional nursing.

In this field of nursing you must have patience, understanding, observational skills, and current first-aid techniques and principles. You must possess organizational skills and neatness in keeping records. You must be able to adjust to all types of situations and people.

◆ The Licensed Practical Nurse in Private Duty Nursing

As a private duty nurse you may care for your patient wherever the patient desires. This may be in the home, the hospital, or while traveling abroad or in the United States. In this field you are given the opportunity to know your patient and his family better. You will be expected to meet the total needs of the patient. This includes rendering bedside care if needed, showering him with attention, and catering to his every whim and fancy unless contraindicated. You not only accept the patient when doing private duty nursing, but his family as well. Many times the patient's problems become your problems. Teaching the patient and his family may be one of your chief functions.

When doing private duty nursing, you are legally responsible for your own actions. If you should experience any doubt about an order or procedure, obtain clarification from the physician before carrying out the order or procedure. Careful charts must be kept. In a hospital setting use the procedure of the hospital. In the home set up a type of record in which you can list necessary items, such as medications given, vital signs, and the condition of the patient. This home record may be requested by the patient's physician and may be released by you to him. Remember that any narcotics not used must be returned to the physician before you leave the case.

The salary scale set by the licensed practical nurse associations and by the American Nurses' Association is approximately three-fourths the salary of the registered nurse for 8 hours of duty.

The chief problems of a private duty nurse are the irregular assignments and the economic aspects. In private duty nursing there is no certainty of an available case or of payment. However, because today there are so many unfilled demands for private duty nurses, the availability of cases presents few problems for the licensed practical nurse. The greater problem centers around payment. The patient is responsible for the payment of the fee even if a member of the family hires the nurse. The family is not legally responsible for the payment of the fee. Therefore fees are occasionally difficult to collect.

If you should choose this field of nursing, it is advisable to remember that you will be responsible for the payment of your social security, as well as your federal, state, and city taxes. This means that you must keep continuous, accurate records of your days worked and payments received.

An advantage of private duty nursing is that you may work as many days as you like, or you may not accept a case for as long a period of time as you desire. You are given more freedom and less rigid rules to follow in your workday.

◆ The Licensed Practical Nurse in the General Hospital

There are many opportunities available in the hospital to use your abilities as a licensed practical nurse to the fullest extent. If giving direct care to the patient is your greatest interest, then working as a bedside nurse will meet your needs. Often by working directly with the patient, you become the most important person in the hospital to him. You spend longer periods of time with him than any of the other personnel. You can help meet the patient's needs by accurately reporting them to the team leader or head nurse, who in turn will report them to the physician. Your duties will depend on hospital policies and your training and work record. You should be familiar with the hospital's job description for the position for which you have been employed. A careful study of this job description will clearly define your role in the health team.

The 8-hour tour of duty that you will follow will usually be 7 AM to 3:30 PM, 3 PM to 11:30 PM, or 11 PM to 7:30 AM. It may be any one of these, or it may be a combination of all of these. Usually your days off will be rotated so that everyone will have equal opportunity for holidays and weekends. Before accepting a position, you should check and know the hospital's policies concerning tours of duty. This will help you to make previous arrangements so that you can follow duty schedules.

There are many advantages to working in a hospital. Employment is steady, and most hospitals have good personnel policies. Ordinarily you can choose any one of the specific areas in the hospital that are available. These areas include obstetrics, pediatrics, general medicine, surgery, and psychiatry. They may also include one of the specialties such as the operating room.

Nurses will choose to work in the clinical area that best fits their personalities, skills, and needs. For instance, did you ever notice the typical nurse in a surgical area? Usually the operating room nurse is quick moving, energetic, and adept with machines and procedures. In the surgical area there is always the high dramatic element: the psychological preparation before surgery and the first critical postoperative hours with much pain and possible complications, usually followed by dramatic daily improvement. Nausea, distention, and inability to void are common postoperative problems. Various drainage tubes, chest tube bottles, tracheostomy care, and dressing changes create a challenging environment and warrant an observing practitioner skilled at working in such a situation. The surgical nurse may communicate more with actions than words.

Contrast the surgery patient to the patient in a coronary care unit whose wound is not visible although he is possibly in more imminent danger of death. A coronary patient requires a nurse with a particular emotional makeup, depth of knowledge, and the ability to recognize subtle signs of a changing condition. This nurse must be able to recognize a multitude of monitor patterns and be able to act quickly and expertly without alarming the patient. It is a demanding role that requires a certain equanimity and type of personality.

Medical nursing is challenging because of the subtlety of signs, changing conditions, and the necessity of sustaining the spirit of patients with long, often chronic, recurring exacerbations of their illness; it requires a nurse who has great empathy and endurance.

A good psychiatric nurse must have a stable emotional makeup. Because so much of psychiatric nursing involves active therapy for the depressed and apathetic patient, this is not an area for the overly empathetic and emotional nurse. Although there is little physical expenditure in psychiatric nursing, there is much mental strain and tension.

Some nurses like to function in extremely active areas with little time for rest and relaxation such as in the emergency room, delivery room, or treatment room. The night shift in the emergency room may deal with two minor conditions one night and perhaps twenty critical conditions the next night, including a cardiac arrest and five admissions. In all these areas experiences will be varied and offer many opportunities for learning.

While working in a general hospital, you will find opportunities to advance both your knowledge and your skills. The duties you may perform as a licensed practical nurse will be regulated by the state board of nursing as well as by the individual hospital. Regardless of your preparation and experience, you may perform only those procedures and functions legislated for the status of a licensed practical nurse.

All practical nurses working in specialized areas need postgraduate training to better qualify them for the role they are expected to fulfill. In a hospital, this may include a Basic Dysrhythmia course and/or an I.V. Therapy course; in a nursing home, courses in management and leadership; in home health care, courses that help the nurse better develop assessment skills and interpersonal relationships.

The community, the hospital, your professional organizations, and your patients depend on you to continue your education through in-service programs, courses, or readings. Only by keeping abreast of nursing and its newest procedures and theories will you be able to function adequately.

◆ The Licensed Practical Nurse in Other Areas

Licensed practical nurses are employed in fields of nursing other than the four areas just mentioned. However, the number of licensed practical nurses in these areas is considerably smaller. Following are some of these fields.

Office Nursing

Advantages
    Covered by Social Security
    Usually have Sundays and most evenings free
    Holidays, vacations, duties, and salaries are determined by the physician
Disadvantages
    Work includes secretarial knowledge and skills

Rehabilitation Nursing

Employment in rehabilitation requires a nurse who will assume responsibility for guiding the patient toward health and independence.
    Advantages
    Steady employment
    Less formal environment
    An opportunity to provide good bedside care
    Disadvantages
    Frequently faced with greater responsibility than generally, educationally, and
        technically prepared to assume

Extended Care Facilities (ECF)

ECF nursing is care of the patient during the intermediate period when he no longer requires hospital care but is not well enough to go home.

Advantages

Steady employment

Holidays, vacations, duties, and salaries are determined by the institution

Greater opportunity for advancement

Disadvantages

Poorer salaries and benefits

Frequently faced with greater responsibility than generally, educationally, and technically prepared to assume

Nursing Homes

Work in a convalescent (nursing) home requires a mature nurse with a genuine interest and liking for geriatric nursing.

Advantages

Less formal environment

Hours usually more stable

Greater opportunity for advancement

Disadvantages

Occasionally substandard patient care

Poorer salaries and working conditions

Frequently faced with greater responsibility than generally, educationally, and technically prepared to assume

Psychiatric Nursing

Psychiatric nursing requires a mature person (not in years) to handle the responsibilities of the job. This type of nursing may be done in an open ward in a general hospital, outpatient clinic, mental health agency, psychiatric hospital, or institution.

Advantages

Good salary

Advancement in leadership areas

Disadvantages

If federally financed, often poorer standard of patient care and working conditions

Insufficient professional guidance from nursing staff and physician

Home Health Care

Employment in home health nursing requires a nurse who will assume responsibility for giving nursing care and guiding the patient toward health and independence. This care may be offered by hospitals, governments, or private organizations.

Advantages

Steady employment

Less formal environment

Opportunities to assess and provide patient needs

Disadvantages
  Can care for very ill patients in a home setting
  Less equipment than would be available in a hospital
  May travel to more than one home each shift

Hospice Care

Employment in hospice nursing requires a mature person (not in years) to meet the spiritual, physical, emotional, and social needs of the dying person and his family. This type of nursing may be done in a hospital, another facility, or the patient's home.
  Advantages
    Steady employment
    Less formal environment
    Opportunities to provide good bedside care that is concerned with pain relief
      and comfort measures
  Disadvantages
    Always caring for dying patients
    May travel to more than one home each shift

Government

Civil service. The licensed practical nurse may work in a Veterans Administration hospital or other government hospital.
  Advantages
    Good salary
    Fringe benefits
    Good insurance and retirement plans
  Disadvantages
    The ratio of nursing personnel to patients is sometimes low

Agency. Agency nurses must be flexible and willing to follow the policies and procedures of many institutions.
  Advantages
    Can choose days and shifts you want to work
    Good salary
  Disadvantages
    Must work in many different institutions
    May not have benefits such as sick leave and insurance included

Armed services (army). The army requires the licensed practical nurse to be between 17 and 34 years of age and a United States citizen of high moral and personal qualifications. The nurse must be a graduate of a 1-year practical nursing program and currently licensed.
  Advantages
    Patriotic service to country
    Travel
    Varied experiences are usually encountered

Special rank and pay

Allowance given for clothing and quarters

Benefits of education, training, medical and dental care, and survivors' insurance

Disadvantages

Varied shifts and often rotating divisions

Regimented type of life

◆ The Licensed Practical Nurse and Public Relations

In your daily work in the nursing field you will come into close contact with many classifications of workers. All these workers contribute to the patient's welfare either directly or indirectly. They include the physician, registered nurse, student nurse, and ancillary personnel such as nursing assistant and the other members of the health team spread throughout the hospital. Cooperation, kindness, and friendliness must exist among all workers to create a successful healing environment for the patient.

You will also be an important representative of the hospital to your patients and their families.

Physicians

Physicians are the direct link between the patient and the members of the health team. Their orders should be carried out as written; if you have any doubt concerning their interpretation or accuracy, you should ask the physician in a diplomatic way how the order should be executed because you are legally liable for your actions. Always be courteous and cooperative. While on duty do not become overly familiar with physicians. Do not ask for free medical service or discuss personal problems with them during working hours. Use physicians' last names when speaking to them.

Inspire the patient by showing confidence in his physician. The patient chose his own physician; therefore this choice should be respected. Never suggest to the patient that he can change physicians or ask for consultation from another physician. If you believe that something should be done about the patient's physician, discuss the matter with your head nurse, who is responsible for the patient's welfare and has had experience in handling this type of situation.

Registered Nurses

In a hospital you will be working under the supervision of a registered nurse, who retains authority because of advanced training and education. Registered nurses and practical nurses, together with other ancillary personnel, work as a team providing optimum patient care. Much can be accomplished on a busy nursing unit and in a lesser amount of time if registered nurses and practical nurses work together, each respecting the other's expertise, work experience, and maturity.

If problems arise, team members should be able to discuss them intelligently and arrive at an acceptable solution. In this manner, each will grow, each will learn to depend on the other, and the result will be a more harmonious, more efficient nursing division. It is essential to remember that one can always learn, that trust is earned, and that respect is the desire of all. One of the best ways to earn respect is to do a job well.

Student Nurses

If you are working in a hospital where there are student nurses, from either the professional or the practical nursing program, remember that the objectives are the same for all—"good nursing care." There may be various ways of carrying out a procedure, but the underlying principles of the procedure never change. Always use proper technique when performing any duty, procedure, or function. Proper technique is the greatest assurance of protection for the patient. In the event that you see a student or registered nurse performing a procedure that is neither correct for the patient nor in the best interest of the hospital, report this immediately to your instructor or charge nurse, who will check into the matter and make the necessary corrections.

Ancillary Personnel

It is never professional to brag or boast about your accomplishments. You may be better prepared than others with whom you are working. However, this should be an incentive for you to assist your fellow workers in any way possible. Never use a condescending attitude. If a co-worker has made an error and it is your responsibility to correct him, then do so in the proper manner. Call the person aside to assure privacy, and correct him in a constructive manner. If the error continues, then report the matter to the charge nurse or head nurse.

In working with nonnursing members of the health team, always remember that these personnel have their respective supervisors who are responsible for them. Any incident or error you believe needs reporting should be reported to your charge nurse, who in turn will follow the proper lines of authority to remedy the situation. Only in an emergency would you have the right to correct another hospital employee. Common sense should be used in this type of situation.

You can win acceptance, respect, and admiration from all with whom you work by doing your job efficiently and thoroughly. This includes being cooperative, understanding, and courteous at all times.

Patients

You can be an important public relations person for the hospital. The patient has so many needs to be met while he is sick that to meet these needs adequately you must acquire as much information as possible concerning both his physical and mental needs. Every patient has certain capacities, interests, and desires. These are influenced by his socioeconomic background, religion, and personal and work experiences. You must know how his illness will alter or affect his attitudes and behavior.

While caring for the patient's physical needs, you must recognize the emotional needs created by this illness. Because humans are complex, physical and mental needs cannot be treated separately. They interact with each other; therefore they must be treated simultaneously.

Many patients find inactivity difficult. This fact is particularly true if the patient was very active before his illness. Given more time for thinking, he often develops many fears and tends to worry excessively. At times you may be able to alleviate some of these worries and fears. A simple explanation concerning procedures to be performed, an understanding attitude, and taking time to listen are some of the ways that you can give the patient the assurance that he may need.

Every patient is different. Some patients may tolerate a great deal of pain, remain optimistic, and require little attention. Others, although they may experience only slight pain, may become easily depressed or require much attention from the nursing staff. The patient's forced state of helplessness may cause him to react differently from his normal state of behavior. He may hesitate to make his needs known. He may not respond to a cheerful atmosphere. He may require a serious approach. Some patients want to talk about their condition; others will shy away from the subject. You must be alert to detect the patient's response and treat each patient accordingly.

You must be able to convey in some manner, either by words or actions, that you are trying to help the patient. All of your actions, the time that you spend with him, and the procedures that you must perform are done to help remedy or alleviate his present diseased condition. Unless you are able to convince the patient of this help, you will not gain his cooperation, and his condition may not improve. He must have confidence in you if you are to be effective. You must have tolerance, personal self-control, and an understanding of his difficulties. Your best approach to any patient is a positive, wholesome attitude.

With a heavy work assignment and the continuing shortage of personnel in many areas, you may find it difficult to take time to listen to your patient's problems. However, allowing the patient to express his feelings may prove to be the best type of therapy. If you merely listen in a hurried manner and tell him not to worry, you have accomplished nothing for him. The patient wants to know that you understand his problems, are interested in them, and will find a solution for them if at all possible. When dealing with other people's problems, you are not emotionally involved and therefore can be more objective than they. Console the patient as much as you can, in view of your understanding of his attitudes and problems.

Although a person may complain a great deal, he usually will not reveal his real worries. You should not pry into your patient's personal life, but you may ask encouraging questions that may help your patient to reveal his real problems. If you can help him to achieve a positive attitude toward solving these problems, you have given him the courage to hope again. Without hope, little can be accomplished.

Families

You must exercise tact and have a good understanding of human nature to deal with the families of your patients. They are entrusting you, a stranger, with the care of their loved one. They want to have confidence in you, but you must instill this feeling in them.

It is difficult for families to behave normally during the serious illness of a relative. Some families become excited and highly emotional during this time. You can alleviate some of a family's apprehension by listening to their suggestions concerning the likes and dislikes of the patient in matters of food and personal care. If these suggestions do not interfere with the physician's orders, it may prove helpful to follow them.

Any reassurance that you show to the family serves as an indirect means of helping your patient to develop a good attitude toward you and the care you are giving to him. The family and the patient must believe that you are really interested. Nursing is not just a job to be done but rather a service to be given to your fellow man.

◆ *Study Helps*

1. List the duties of a licensed practical nurse in public health. What are some of the school health services offered by the public health department?
2. What requisites are necessary for licensed practical nurses working in industry? What are their duties?
3. Explain some of the special problems encountered by a licensed practical nurse while doing private duty nursing. Who regulates salaries?
4. List the advantages available to the licensed practical nurse working in a general hospital.
5. Explain the relationship that should exist between the licensed practical nurse and the physician and the licensed practical nurse and the registered nurse.
6. What should the licensed practical nurse's attitude be toward student nurses?
7. Describe how the licensed practical nurse can work effectively with ancillary personnel.
8. Explain the patient's reaction to illness. What is the responsibility of the licensed practical nurse in this area?
9. Explain the family's reaction to illness. What can the licensed practical nurse do to help them?
10. List the advantages available to the licensed practical nurse working for an agency.

Bibliography

Abruzzese RS et al: Practices, ed 1, Springhouse, Pennsylvania, 1984, Springhouse Book Co.
Douglass LM: The effective nurse, ed 3, St Louis, 1988, The CV Mosby Co.
Grippando GM: Nursing perspectives and issues, ed 2, New York, 1983, Delmar Publishers Inc.
Jaffe MS and Skidmore-Roth L: Home health nursing care plans, St Louis, 1988, The CV Mosby Co.
Mason MA and Bates GF: Basic medical-surgical nursing, ed 5, New York, 1984, Macmillan Co.

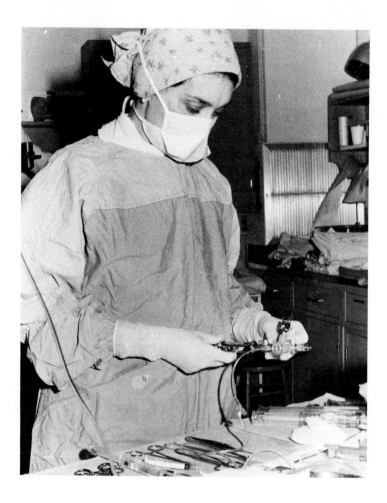

Objectives

At the completion of this chapter the student practical nurse
will be able to:

- Discuss self-evaluation.
- List important benefits when seeking employment.
- Develop a personal budget plan.
- Discuss ways in which an individual can continue his education.
- Differentiate between BSN, ADN, and diploma nursing
  programs.

10 Entry Into Practice and Continuing Education

In all probability you will seek and accept a position of employment in nursing even before you have received your license to practice. However, doing so is permissible because the state board of nursing allows you to work 30 to 90 days, depending on the individual state, while you are applying for and receiving your licensure.

Your choice of employment should be considered carefully. You should be familiar with the fields open to the licensed practical nurse. You should know yourself. Self-knowledge includes knowing your abilities and skills, likes and dislikes, strengths and weaknesses. You must also consider the personal and professional satisfaction that you hope to gain from this specific type of job.

◆ Self-Evaluation

Self-evaluation means examining one's assets as well as one's defects. Two points that should always be included are self-sufficiency and self-confidence. The rule of success is "have a positive attitude and know yourself."

You cannot function well in every area. Your likes and dislikes influence your performance. Your instructors can be of great assistance in helping you to select a suitable and enjoyable field in which to work. The instructors, through learning and experience, are in a position to evaluate your capabilities. Through periodic conferences and counseling they aim to help you strengthen your weak areas and develop your strong areas. Listen to suggestions from those who know you and want to help you. Perhaps they can open new horizons that you have never considered. Accept criticism gracefully and profit from it. You do not have to agree with it, but try to be realistic and honest with yourself. A careful study of your personality, your abilities, and your achievements in nursing will help you to decide the area of nursing for which you are best suited. Your aim is to fulfill the needs of others, but in doing so you must fulfill certain needs of your own.

◆ Position Analysis

You will not find a perfect job. Each one has advantages and disadvantages. The selection of a field of nursing is a major decision. Previously, licensed practical nurses had few areas from which to choose; today there are many fields that they may enter. Remember that every field will not appeal to everyone. Humans were not created with the same likes and dislikes, the same personalities, or the same beliefs. If interests vary, then the type of work suited to each person will also vary.

A quick look at some of the advantages and disadvantages in the major areas available to the practical nurse today may prove beneficial.

Finding a Position

There is a shortage of nursing personnel in some areas. You may discover available positions through word of mouth, hospitals, schools, agencies, or advertisements. Because the qualifications for the job, the benefits, and the possible drawbacks can be easily distorted, never presume. Know the full responsibilities, the salary, and the hours. Ask to see the personnel policies and read them carefully. Arrange for a personal interview before you make any commitments.

Evaluation of Positions

When evaluating positions, many factors must be considered. Some of these factors include salary, hours and days, vacation and sick leave, maternity leave, adoptive leave, child care, leave of absence and holiday time, transportation, reputation of employer, promotional opportunities, laundry and uniforms, meals, in-service education, environmental factors, and insurance benefits. Each of these factors will be discussed briefly. Ask yourself questions concerning each of the following considerations.

Salary. Salary is important, but it is not everything. Other factors such as opportunities for advancement, experience, further educational opportunities, and increments after you have proved your worth are also important. Sometimes high salaries are offered because the position requires more responsibility than you as a practical nurse are prepared to assume. High salaries are often used as an enticement to secure nurses for needed positions. Although a good salary is important, equally important is a good benefits package; *both* factors should be considered when seeking employment.

Hours and days. Are you planning to work full time or part time? What hours are entailed? Must you rotate shifts? How many weekends must you work?

Vacation and sick leave. Two benefits are vacation and sick time. Ask yourself these questions: Is a time for sick leave and vacation provided? If so, how long is it? Is it with or without pay? Does it increase with the length of service? Does the hospital give a discount for room and medications if needed by the employee?

Maternity leave. Does the institution provide time off for the birth of a baby? If so, how long?

Adoptive leave. Does the institution provide time off for the mother of an adoptive child? How long?

Child care. Does the institution provide child care for its employees? If so, what are the hours, the cost, and the ages of children accepted? Are the people employed to care for the children dependable, knowledgeable, and caring? Is the facility near a part of the hospital to which you are applying?

Leave of absence and holiday time. How many holidays are provided each year? Is a leave of absence granted? If so, which conditions are necessary to obtain this leave? Is it with or without pay? What is the employee's status on returning from a leave?

Transportation. How far is the institution from where you live? Do you have a car? If not, is there adequate bus service available? Can you really depend on another person for transportation? Will rotation of shifts cause transportation problems? Are there free, safe, and adequate parking facilities?

Reputation of employer. Does the employer or institution have a good reputation? Is it known for its high standards? Is it accredited by professional organizations? Is the turnover of nursing personnel high? If so, investigate this turnover thoroughly.

Promotional opportunities. Are periodic raises given? Are they automatic, or are they dependent on a personal evaluation of your performance? What is the top salary that is available to a licensed practical nurse? What length of time is normally required to obtain it?

Laundry and uniforms. Must you supply or launder your own uniforms, or will the institution provide this service? Which types of uniforms are allowed? Which uniform regulations exist for the employee?

Meals. Do the employees receive free meals while on duty? If not, do they receive a discount? Are coffee breaks provided? If so, how many are there and for what length of time? Does the institution have a cafeteria or suitable place in which to eat?

In-service education. Is the institution education minded? Is there an orientation program? Is there a program for in-service education? Which areas are covered by the program? How often are these programs given?

Tuition reimbursement. Does the institution offer tuition reimbursement to employees desiring to continue their education outside the hospital? Must the courses be job related? Is this benefit available upon employment or after a time of employment? How much of the tuition cost will be reimbursed to the employee? If this education is college related, how many credit hours may the employee take in one semester? Must the employee achieve a certain grade to be reimbursed? How long a time may the employee take to achieve his educational goal?

Environmental factors. Is the institution neat, clean, cheerful, and progressive? Is it equipped with the up-to-date machinery that is needed to render quality nursing care to the patient? What is the morale of the employees?

Insurance benefits. Does the institution make provisions for group or individual plans? Which types of insurance plans does it offer—life, liability, salary continuance, medical, and dental plans? What is the coverage of these insurance plans? Does the employer carry compensation insurance for accidents or sickness of the employee?

If the institution does not provide liability insurance, the practical nurse should think in terms of securing it to cover claims as well as costs of legal counsel that may arise from negligence or damage or both occurring while giving care. With liability insurance you are covered even if the claim is false, groundless, or fraudulent. The premiums are deductible from your federal income tax. Group premium rates are available through most state licensed practical nurse associations. The constantly increasing number of lawsuits involving alleged malpractice now makes liability insurance a necessity.

Credit union. Does the institution have a credit union? Is the employee able to make a deposit in a credit union account through a payroll deduction? How much interest is paid to the investor? How much interest is charged by the credit union for a personal loan?

Pension plan. Who is eligible? Does the employer pay the premium, or is a portion deducted from the employee's paycheck? What percentage of base pay will the employee receive on retirement? Is there a compulsory retirement age?

◇   ◇   ◇

After you have thoroughly evaluated these factors, you must decide whether the position is suitable for you, both personally and economically.

◆ Applying for a Position

After you have carefully considered the type of position you want and its various aspects, you must apply for the position. This can be done by written application or by personal interview. If you are applying by written application, keep the essentials of good letter writing in mind. Use white paper. Never use colored or lined paper. Either type your letter or write it in ink. Use the proper salutation. Avoid using the phrase "to whom it may concern." Use proper English, spell correctly, and use correct punctuation. Provide margins on your letter. Do not enclose photographs, diplomas, or references unless specified. When you wish to use a person's name as a reference, ask the person for permission to use his name. Be sure to thank him for the reference. A sample letter is shown on p. 141.

The following points should be included in your letter:
1. State the purpose of the letter and the position for which you are applying.

◆ *Sample Letter of Application*

3900 North Plane St.
St. Louis, MO 63104
January 5, 1989

Ms. Joan Price R.N.
Director of Nurses
Barnes Hospital
One Barnes Hospital Plaza
St. Louis, MO 63110

Dear Ms. Price:

I would appreciate your consideration of me as an applicant for the position of licensed practical nurse you advertised in today's copy of the *St. Louis Post-Dispatch.*

I am a graduate of St. Mary's School of Practical Nursing in St. Louis, Mo. For the past 7 years I have been working as a licensed practical nurse in a general hospital on a surgical division. I have functioned as a team leader, medicine nurse, treatment nurse, and, on occasion, a charge nurse.

May I have an appointment for an interview at your earliest convenience? You may write to the above address or call me at 876-5431 after 5 P.M.

Sincerely yours,

John Ames, L.P.N.

2. Give the source of information concerning the job. This may be through advertisement, a previous employer, or a recommendation from someone.
3. Give your qualifications and past experiences. They will help the employer to judge whether you have the proper preparation for the job.
4. You may request an application blank or an appointment for an interview.
5. Express your appreciation for the employer's consideration.
6. Sign your full name and give your address and phone number.

Application Form

Most places of employment will request you to complete an application form before you are interviewed. These forms may vary with the institution, but all forms essentially contain the following:

Your name (include your maiden name if married)
Address
Telephone number
Social Security number

License number

Education

Previous places of employment, their addresses, and the length of time employed
in each place

Reference names and addresses

Job for which you are applying

An application form aids the employer in eliminating the applicants who do not
possess the desired qualifications for the position and provides the employer with
necessary information. It becomes an important part of the employer's file if the
applicant is hired, or it may be kept on file for future openings requiring these
qualifications.

Interview

Always make an appointment in advance for an interview. This may be done by
letter or by phone. This shows consideration for the employer, and it also assures you of
a specific time and date.

The purpose of the interview is twofold. It provides the employer with the
opportunity to determine whether you qualify for the position, and it gives you the
opportunity to evaluate the job in terms of your needs and expectations. Therefore
both the interviewer and you will have two objectives in mind: giving and receiving
information. Each is evaluating the other.

Be sure to be on time, preferably a few minutes early. Try to be composed and
relaxed. Make sure that you are properly groomed and dressed. Know the name of the
person who is to interview you. Never chew gum! Do not smoke unless invited to do so.
Remain standing until you are told to be seated. Remain poised and alert. Listen
carefully and answer as simply and honestly as possible. Neither exaggerate nor
underestimate your abilities. When asked about your previous experiences, state them
in a matter-of-fact manner.

Before you accept the position, be sure that it is the type of position that you are
seeking and desire. Know the salary, the personnel policies, and the duties and responsibilities that will be expected of you. If several people are applying for the same
position, ask the interviewer when he plans to make a decision. If you do not believe
that the position is suited to you, then express these feelings to the interviewer. Thank
him for his time and interest and leave.

♦ Retaining Your Position

To retain your position you must accept its imposed responsibilities. This includes
reporting on and off duty, notifying the proper person if ill, and giving your employer
sufficient time to secure a replacement. You should understand your duties and show
interest in their performance. Be willing to give the best of your abilities and show their
worth to others. Above all, try to find happiness and success in your job. All jobs have
good and bad points, but usually the good points outweigh the bad. Do not change jobs
too frequently. Recommendations are better the longer you retain a certain position.
Never walk away from your duties or responsibilities. Remember that in return for

your services the employer has contracted to pay you a definite salary with certain fringe benefits. He has a right to demand a good day's work in return for a just salary. If you take a strong character and a good personality to a new position, you will advance both personally and professionally. Joy in what you are doing, together with sufficient preparation and knowledge, will help you to give quality nursing care to the patient and be a pleasant co-worker to members of the team.

Advancement

Advancement may result from additional preparation or additional experience. It may be made by learning the position more thoroughly and by assuming new and greater responsibilities. Advancements, together with the difficulties and obstacles that they bring, stimulate interest and enthusiasm. They are usually based on a person's qualifications, behavior, performance, and preparation.

Resignations

If you should decide to resign your position in a certain institution, think the matter over carefully. After you have reached your decision, give at least a 2-week notice, depending on personnel policies of the institution. Never walk off duty without previous notice. In rare circumstances the notice may be shortened or omitted with legitimate reasons. A sample letter of resignation is shown below. Some institutions

---

◆ *Sample Letter of Resignation*

February 9, 1989

Ms. Marsha Hunt
Director of Nurses
Deaconess Hospital
6150 Oakland Avenue
St. Louis, MO 63139

Dear Ms. Hunt:

I am resigning my position as a medical nurse. My husband has been transferred to another state, and the move will require much of my time.

I am giving the mandatory 2-week notice. My last day will be February 23, 1989.

It has been a pleasure to work here for the past 5 years. I have made many friends and am grateful to you and to the staff for the many opportunities and the assistance I have received.

Sincerely yours,

Eloise Just, L.P.N.

have typed resignation forms to be filled in by the employee. These forms include the date of termination, reasons for leaving, and evaluation of employment. Make arrangements for your final paycheck. Take the resignation form or letter to your employer in person if possible. Leave the institution in good standing; keep any feelings of resentment to yourself. Remember that future recommendations depend on your manner and procedure of resignation.

Dismissals

Reasons for dismissals may be dishonesty, insubordination, unlawful or wrong actions, or failure to observe rules and regulations. In these instances you may be discharged without notice and may forfeit any benefits such as holidays, sick leave, or vacation time. You will be paid in full for the days worked. In most cases of dismissal a 2-week notice is given. If you believe that the dismissal is unfair, you have the right to appeal to the director of personnel. The director has the duty to hear and review your case and make the final decision. If dismissal occurs during the probationary period or from a temporary position, you are not entitled to any benefits. Dismissal policies may vary in different types of institutions.

Failure

Why do some people fail in their positions? Sometimes failure may be attributed to character limitations. These limitations may include poor interpersonal relationships, lack of cooperation, insincerity, and jealousy. Other causes of failure may be lack of knowledge regarding the position, inability to deal with patients and co-workers, or failure to demonstrate one's abilities. Every employee has basic needs that must be fulfilled. Recognition and acceptance are important needs that must be met. If they are not met, job dissatisfaction and insecurity may result.

The type of position you choose must meet your needs, and you must meet the needs of the job. If the position you choose fails to bring you satisfaction, you will be unhappy and your behavior and patient care will soon reflect this. If you are unprepared for the position you choose, you will soon experience frustration and be overwhelmed by the expectations of your employer. What can you do? There are two alternatives: change positions or do something to correct the problem. If you feel the job does not meet your needs and you can do nothing to effect a change, resignation would be your alternative. If you feel educationally unprepared, consider continuing your education. A wise person never stops learning, and learning can be attained in many ways: learning on the job, in-service programs in the hospital, attending conventions and workshops, reading professional journals, watching educational television programs, or taking regular or extension courses in a postgraduate school, college, or junior college. The most important factor is your willingness to change and to learn. Regardless of the types of educational programs made available to you, they will be of little or no value unless you want to learn.

◆ Budget

Your economic status determines the way you live. Therefore the wise spending of money necessitates a budget.

Suggested Budget Plan

A budget or spending plan is a tool. It helps you to manage money wisely and to attain your financial goals. A budget can help you eliminate inefficient spending and give you more for your money. To be workable, your budget must be tailored for you. It should be adapted to your needs and income. Preparing a budget for yourself takes planning, and following a budget requires determination.

There are all types of forms and systems for handling money, but the principle is still the same. You must list your definite obligations and in this way discover how much money you must put aside to meet these future outlays. From this you will be able to estimate how much money you have to spend from day to day and how much you will be able to save.

In its simplest form a money management plan consists of four sets of figures. It makes little difference with which set you begin. For convenience the sets have been assigned a certain order and labeled Steps 1, 2, 3, and 4 (p. 146). The following plan is based on a weekly system. You will be asked to determine items on an annual basis and divide by 52. If you prefer to use a semimonthly or monthly basis, you will divide by 24 or 12 rather than 52.

Step 1: your income. Write down how much money you expect to receive in a 12-month period. Be certain to include all types of income. Add these items and divide by 52. This will be your weekly income. When listing wages and salaries, write down what you will actually be receiving. Do not include withholding taxes and other types of deductions. This does not mean, however, that it is safe for you to ignore payroll deductions when you establish your program. If a deduction is for hospitalization or group life insurance, it is a payment toward your protection. If it is for the purchase of a savings bond or a pension, it is a payment toward your savings. Some payroll deductions are set by law. Others can be increased or decreased as your situation changes.

Step 2: your weekly set-asides. Write down all the fixed obligations you will have to meet during a 12-month period. Examples of these are rent or mortgage payments, installment payments, life insurance, church contributions, and taxes over and above your payroll tax. It may help if you indicate which month these outlays are due. Do not write down expenses you cannot estimate closely, but do not include fixed obligations or expenses you can estimate. Total these fixed items, then divide by 52. The answer you receive will be what you set aside weekly. Each week you must put this amount in the bank or a special fund; when one of your fixed items comes due, pay it from this fund. Once the system is well under way, if your original estimates were correct, there will always be sufficient funds to meet your obligations.

Step 3: your emergency fund. To make your financial plan work and to meet unexpected future expenses, you will need a reserve fund. It need not be a large sum of money but enough to tide you over bad weeks or months. Take care not to confuse your emergency fund with savings. The purpose of the emergency fund is not for advancement, to purchase something in the future, or a provision for long-term security. It is a fund to tide you over temporary emergencies. Be conservative when estimating how

◆ *Sample Budget*

Step 1: your income

1.	Take-home pay	Annual	$15000.00
		Weekly	288.46

Step 2: your weekly set-asides

1.	Rent (shared)	Annual	2000.00
2.	Payment on car	Annual	1800.00
3.	Contributions (church, United Fund, etc.)	Annual	85.00
4.	Life insurance	Annual	250.00
5.	Car insurance	Annual	650.00
		Annual total	4785.00
		Weekly total (divided by 52)	92.02

Step 3: your emergency fund

	Annual	700.00
	Weekly	13.46

Step 4: your living expenses

1.	Food (shared)	Annual	2000.00
2.	Utilities (shared)	Annual	400.00
3.	Clothing	Annual	1000.00
4.	Car maintenance (gas, oil, repairs)	Annual	1500.00
5.	Medical-dental expenses	Annual	400.00
6.	Personal allowances	Annual	800.00
		Annual total	6100.00
		Weekly total (divided by 52)	117.30

Savings: Add annual expenses of Steps 2, 3, and 4. Subtract total from annual income. Result is *annual savings*.

Add weekly expenses of Steps 2, 3, and 4. Subtract total from weekly income. Result is *weekly savings*.

large a fund you will need. Some people suggest 1 month's, 2 months', or 3 months' income, but that must be a decision based on what you know your needs will be. When you have figured the amount to be put in your emergency fund, write it down and add it to the amount you set aside weekly. Every week put this money into a special fund or bank account. When you believe your emergency fund is large enough, stop putting money in it. Instead, increase your regular savings program, life insurance, or investments, or use the money in some other way.

Step 4: your living expenses. Take your weekly income, subtract the allowance for your emergency fund and the amount you set aside weekly, and arrive at a weekly figure with which to pay your day-to-day expenses. These are clothing, food, utilities, transportation, car maintenance, personal allowances, recreation, and other such items. To know if your plan will work, you must estimate these items as closely as possible, then check the total with the amount you estimated for them. If the amount is insufficient, you must refigure the provision you made for other items. The amount remaining after expenses will be your regular savings. Your savings will determine your rate of progress toward reaching your future financial goal.

◆ Continuing Education

In-Service Education

Many hospitals, as well as other places of employment, have in-service education programs. When you secure a new position, the first in-service education that you will probably receive is a program of orientation. If specific procedures must be performed, a series of concentrated classes may follow. An example of such an institution may be a rehabilitation hospital. Although the licensed practical nurse may already be familiar with range of motion exercises, these and other pertinent procedures will be reviewed with new personnel.

Each hospital has its own definite nursing care procedures, and personnel are required to follow these techniques rather than those previously learned. This uniformity helps to assure safety to both patients and personnel. Some institutions provide follow-up classes to keep their employees abreast of current trends in patient care. Other types of in-service educational programs include special classes in the administration of medicines, operating room techniques, labor and delivery care, and cardiopulmonary resuscitation.

These classes are given on duty time. Since they are offered for the advancement of the employee, you should take advantage of them. There should never be a need to force you to attend these classes. Financially it is costly to the institution to offer such programs, but the advances made in nursing care as a result compensate for this cost. If you fail to attend these programs, it is a loss to you, your patients, and the institution where you are employed.

Conventions and Workshops

Conventions and workshops are held locally, statewide, regionally, and nationally in a variety of forms. They may be offered or sponsored by alumni organizations, state organizations, the National Association for Practical Nurse Education and Service, Inc., or the National Federation of Licensed Practical Nurses. There are also 1- to 3-day workshops offered by the American Heart Association and the National Cancer Society. You cannot expect to attend every convention offered. However, if the hospital does not make provision for its employees to attend these conventions or workshops, you may attend them on your day off or request days of your vacation time for this purpose. Programs offered on a local level are usually of shorter duration, and attendance presents fewer problems. You have heard many times that "nothing stands still." Either a person progresses or regresses. The same is true in the nursing profession. Every day new advances, techniques, and methods of nursing care are being developed. Unless you become familiar with these developments and adopt them according to the policies of your hospital or institution, you will gradually become less efficient, and your activities will be limited.

Professional Journals and Publications

Reading articles from professional journals can be very valuable to you. Some are published especially for the licensed practical nurse, including the *Journal of Practical Nursing, Journal of Nursing Care,* and state and local publications.

The *Journal of Practical Nursing* is published by the National Association for Practical Nurse Education and Service, Inc., 254 West 31st Street, New York, NY 10001. It is a monthly publication that will keep you informed about national activities in your practical nursing group. It contains articles on nursing topics, coming events, available positions, new books and pamphlets, and activities occurring in the various states.

The *Journal of Nursing Care* is published by Health Science Division, Technomic Publishing Co., Inc., 265 Post Road West, Westport, CT 06880. It is a monthly publication that contains information about and activities of the National Federation of Licensed Practical Nurses (NFLPN). It includes reports from committees representing practical nursing, progress of practical nursing education programs, and any announcements the national headquarters desires to convey to its members, state or local.

You should become familiar with your state and local nursing publications. They are usually in the form of bulletins, journals, or magazines. They contain valuable information concerning the officers of your state and local divisions of your organization, plus events, programs, achievements, and happenings in your immediate vicinity.

Because procedures and techniques may change with new developments in medicine, you should maintain proficiency by periodically reading new texts and references by leading publishers in nursing. New publications are advertised in most professional journals.

Postgraduate Programs

Postgraduate programs may be very beneficial to a graduate who does not feel adequately prepared to assume responsibilities in a particular field. Some instructors and administrative personnel believe that it is wise for a new graduate to work for 6 months to 1 year in a general hospital to gain necessary experience. During student days some practical experience is acquired, but theory is emphasized. After graduation limited theoretical knowledge is gained, and emphasis is placed on practical experience. After a year spent in a general hospital, the licensed practical nurse has sufficient background to specialize in one particular area and is equipped with a varied background sufficient for functioning smoothly and efficiently.

Before enrolling in a postgraduate program, investigate to see if it is an accredited program. You must consider all factors involved. Some of these include length of time, cost, and living expenses needed. Some programs may mean living away from home or even in another state.

The postgraduate programs available can be found in monthly publications from your local, state, or national organizations. They will list the courses offered, the dates, and the locations where they will be offered.

Refresher Courses

Nursing organizations. Refresher courses are courses offered by the home nursing school, local organizations, or state and national nursing organizations. They are offered to those wishing to bring themselves up-to-date with current trends in nursing care. The length of the course may vary with individual groups, material being taught, and different instructors. Many schools of practical nursing are now offering courses to their alumni and to other interested licensed practical nurses. The most commonly offered course is administration of medicines.

Local branches of the American National Red Cross offer courses such as first aid, swimming, and water safety. The procedures taught in these courses are current and serve as valuable aids to both nursing and nonnursing persons.

Television. Television is being used to give extension courses in useful subjects for continuing education. Many of these programs award certificates on the completion of the course. Notices of these programs can be found in the daily newspaper and television guides and through your employing hospital or agency. These notices are often posted on the bulletin board or announced at various types of meetings.

Registered Nursing Programs Available

Bachelor of science degree in nursing program—BSN program. The bachelor of science degree program is one that consists of approximately 4 years of university or college training. At the completion of the program the graduate qualifies to take a licensing examination to become a registered nurse and also receives a bachelor of science degree in nursing from the university or college.

In this type of program nursing theory and skills are incorporated with managerial theory and skills. Stress is placed on understanding the entire patient in depth. This understanding includes physical, social, psychological, religious, and economic aspects. The program delves deeply into human behavior and methods of effectively coping with problem situations.

The student learns the theory and skills of nursing and is given opportunities to function in all capacities of a registered nurse under proper supervision.

This program tends to mature the student in all aspects. The nurse develops socially, physically, and psychologically. This educational program should provide the individual with the poise and competency required of a registered nurse.

Associate degree nursing program—ADN program. The associate degree nursing program is offered by community colleges, colleges, and universities. It is designed to prepare the student to assume the responsibilities related to direct patient care as a member of the health team in hospitals and in community health agencies after graduation.

In some areas the curriculum has been revised to incorporate the career ladder concept. The first-year curriculum includes the minimum requirements necessary for the student to become eligible for licensure as a licensed practical nurse. On the successful completion of the entire curriculum, the student is eligible to take the state board of nursing examination for licensure as a registered nurse.

The clinical experience is limited in this type of program. Emphasis is placed on educational background. Clinical experience is given in several hospitals.

After this 2-year program an internship program may prove valuable to the new graduate. This program may rotate the new graduate through areas of a general hospital, providing the graduate with ample opportunity to integrate theory with clinical experience.

Diploma program in nursing. The diploma program is a type of program offered by a private institution or organization. It combines nursing theory and skills. The curriculum is planned over a specific period to give the student sufficient time in all major areas of nursing. This amount of time enables the student to learn procedures and disease conditions thoroughly in each area. It rotates the student through every job performed by the registered nurse. Emphasis is placed equally on both theory and clinical experience. It prepares a bedside nurse, team leader, treatment nurse, or medication nurse. At the completion of the course the graduate is qualified to take the licensure examination to become a registered nurse and is awarded a diploma from the nursing school.

Regardless of the type of nursing program you choose, the fundamental objective of each is quality nursing care. Each deals with patients, their families, and other members of the health team. As a nurse you must develop all your potentials. This means that you not only meet your own needs but also those of the patient. As a licensed practical nurse you have responsibilities to yourself, your patients, your nursing organization, and your community. Nursing is a vocation of service. Your uniform is the badge showing the vocation you have chosen; wear it proudly as you serve others.

◆ *Study Helps*

1. What factors should be considered when applying for employment?
2. In which way can a budget help you to remain financially stable?
3. Describe the demeanor of an individual applying for a position.
4. What opportunities are available for continuing your education after graduation?
5. Which types of in-service programs do most institutions offer?
6. Of what importance are conventions and workshops?
7. Differentiate among the following: BSN degree nursing programs, ADN nursing programs, and diploma programs.
8. What type of vocation is nursing?

Bibliography

Bullough B, Bullough V, and Soukup MC: Nursing issues and nursing strategies for the eighties, ed 1, New York, 1983, Springer Publishing Co, Inc.

De Young L: Dynamics of nursing, ed 4, St Louis, 1981, The CV Mosby Co.

Howe J et al: The handbook of nursing, ed 1, New York, 1984, John Wiley & Sons, Inc.

Milliken ME and Campbell G: Essential competencies for patient care, ed 1, St Louis, 1984, The CV Mosby Co.

Notter L: Essentials of nursing research, ed 3, New York, 1983, Springer Publishing Co, Inc.

Rambo BJ: Adaptation nursing: assessment and intervention, ed 1, Philadelphia, 1984, WB Saunders Co.

Robinson CH and Weigley ES: Basic nutrition and diet therapy, ed 5, New York, 1984, Macmillan Co.

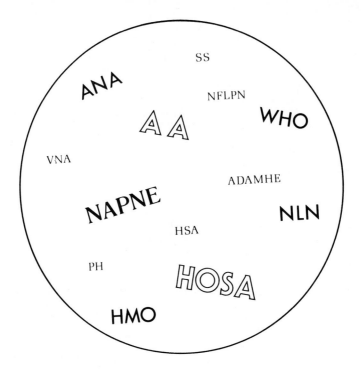

Objectives

At the completion of this chapter the student practical nurse will be able to:

◆ Explain the purposes and function of the Social Security Administration.

◆ List the functions and membership of NAPNES, NFLPN, NLN, and ANA.

◆ List five private and voluntary agencies.

11 Organizations, Insurance, and Agencies

◆ Nursing Organizations

National Association for Practical Nurse Education and Service (NAPNES)

NAPNES (254 West 31st Street, New York, NY 10001), established in 1941, was the first organization for promoting schools of practical nursing and the welfare and continuing education of licensed practical nurses.

In 1959 a new department, the Department of Service to State Practical Nurse Associations, was added; it assists state organizations of practical nursing with any operational and educational problems.

Membership in this organization includes practical nurses, practical nursing students, directors and instructors of schools of practical nursing, nursing home administrators, physicians, professional nurses, and interested lay persons. Membership fees are paid annually either as individual members or through membership in the state association. The subscription to the association's official magazine, the *Journal of Practical Nursing,* is included in the fee. Some of the functions of this organization are as follows:

1. Providing an accrediting program for schools that want to be approved as having met the required standards formulated by NAPNES
2. Providing educational material for faculties to use in practical nursing
3. Issuing guides to those desiring to establish schools of practical nursing
4. Providing a current list of approved schools of practical nursing throughout the country
5. Providing resource personnel for workshops, state conferences, and summer courses for practical nursing educators
6. Recruiting practical nursing students by publicizing and distributing information about practical nursing
7. Collaborating with other nursing organizations in the health field

8. Providing ways for licensed practical nurses to continue their education by sponsoring workshops and encouraging the development and accreditation of postgraduate programs

9. Providing for the welfare of the licensed practical nurse by publishing information about legal aspects of practical nursing, keeping the licensed practical nurse informed about legislation, and sponsoring low-cost group insurance programs

10. Publishing the *Journal of Practical Nursing*

The voting body, which is made up of the constituent state associations, determines the broad policies of the association. The general management responsibility of the association rests with the Board of Directors; the majority of the members are LPNs. Standing committees are assigned many of the activities of the association. These standing committees sometimes delegate tasks to work committees. Provision is made in the bylaws for the formation of councils. Council members are a group of people who have special interests in common.

National Federation of Licensed Practical Nurses, Inc. (NFLPN)

NFLPN (214 S. Driver, P.O. Box 11038, Durham, NC 27703) is the national membership organization and is the policy-making body for licensed practical nurses. NFLPN is the only organization that is composed entirely of licensed practical nurses and serves constituent state associations of like structure. The organization was formed in 1949 by a group of licensed practical nurses to gain status and recognition and to provide an official channel through which licensed practical nurses could speak, act, and work independently on their own behalf.

Membership in this organization is composed of licensed practical nurses and student practical nurses, who may participate in some of the local and state activities. Membership dues are paid once a year; a certain portion of the dues is set aside for national membership dues and the official magazine *The Journal of Nursing Care*. There are two types of membership for the licensed practical nurse; the first are members who join NFLPN through the constituent state association or as a member-at-large. The latter members are those who live in a state that is not a constituent member of NFLPN.

Some functions of this organization are as follows:

1. Concerning itself with the principles of ethics and continuing education for the licensed practical nurse to improve patient care

2. Keeping its members informed concerning matters of interest through the use of letters, bulletins, and appropriate speakers to improve practice

3. Making available to its members health, malpractice, accident, and personal liability insurance plans

4. Working with legislation as the spokesperson on the national level for important matters pertaining to practical nursing

5. Cooperating with other organizations in the health field in the interest of quality and total patient care

6. Continuing to work for licensed practical nurse representation on state boards of nursing

7. Providing a statement of functions and qualifications of the licensed practical nurse that reflects the expanding role of the practical nurse
8. Encouraging all employing agencies to provide in-service education
9. Striving to improve leadership within the organization

In 1972 the NFLPN's House of Delegates passed some major resolutions in the areas of continuing education, standards of licensure, and nursing practice acts. They recommended the study of the concept of mandatory continuing education as a requirement for renewal of a license until such time as an effective method of administration is developed. They recommended that NFLPN go on record as approving the National League for Nursing State Board Test Pool Examination as the standard for licensure. They also recommended that NFLPN support the updating of nursing practice acts to identify licensed practical nurses as peer participants on the professional team responsible for health care delivery and to include the NFLPN definition of practical nursing.

The licensed practical nurse is prepared to function as a member of the health care team by exercising sound nursing judgment based on preparation, knowledge, skills, understanding, and past experiences in nursing situations. But the NFLPN's recommendations show that the practical nurse will have to keep up with rapid changes to meet the increasing responsibilities.

National League for Nursing, Inc. (NLN)

In 1952 the NLN (10 Columbus Circle, New York, NY 10019; branch offices are also in San Francisco and Atlanta) was established by combining programs and resources of three national organizations and four committees. They were the National League for Nursing Education, the Association of Collegiate Schools of Nursing, the National Organization for Public Health Nursing, the Joint Committee on Practical Nurses and Auxiliary Workers in Nursing, the National Committee for the Improvement of Nursing Services, the National Accrediting Service, and the Joint Committee on Careers in Nursing.

NLN membership includes individual members and agency members. An individual member is any person interested in health care and nursing throughout the country. Agency members are nursing schools and nursing services.

NLN has numerous functions that help the nursing profession. It has a department for professional and practical nursing programs. Some functions of this department include the following:

1. Preparing the examination for licensure given to nursing students
2. Accrediting schools of nursing
3. Issuing a current list of scholarships, education grants, and loans for continuing education in the nursing field
4. Informing its members about current issues under evaluation and those newly formulated
5. Cooperating with legislation on the national level in important matters pertaining to nursing
6. Publishing a monthly newsletter that is distributed to all individual and agency members

7. Providing consultation and assistance to programs of nursing as needed
8. Conducting workshops for instructors of schools of nursing throughout the country and providing resource personnel
9. Providing a current list of approved schools of nursing throughout the country
10. Issuing guides to those desiring to establish schools of nursing
11. Providing educational material for use in nursing
12. Publishing *Nursing and Health Care*

The organization is strictly a nursing organization and strives to improve all phases and levels of nursing and nursing care.

NLN Council of Practical Nursing Programs

In 1957 the Council of Practical Nursing Programs was founded. It is concerned with development and improvement of educational programs in practical nursing. The Board of Review for Practical Nursing Programs is appointed by the executive committee and is responsible for evaluating NLN accreditation of practical nursing education. Agency members work together to raise standards and to improve practical nurse preparation within the programs. The Council of Practical Nurse Programs recognizes the need and urges licensed practical nurses to increase their education by taking educational courses that are available.

American Nurses' Association (ANA)

The national organization and official spokesperson for all professional registered nurses is the ANA (2420 Pershing Road, Kansas City, MO 64108), founded in 1896. The ANA is to the professional registered nurse what the NFLPN is to the licensed practical nurse. The membership of this organization is kept informed through its official publications, the *American Journal of Nursing* and *The American Nurse*. The ANA is like the previously discussed nursing organizations in that it works closely with other health and welfare organizations.

Health Occupations Students of America (HOSA)

In 1976 HOSA (New Jersey Department of Education, Division of Vocational Education, 225 West State Street, Trenton, NJ 08625) was founded as a National Vocational Organization. State and local chapters provide activities and programs to help students in health occupations develop their mental, social, and physical well-being. Interactions with student organizations, businesses, and professions strengthen members in leadership and citizenship abilities, in appreciation of helping people, and in developing good decision-making skills. As a practical nursing student, this organization gives you an opportunity to meet students in other health careers and to improve health conditions in the community. For information pertaining to state and local chapters contact your State Department of Education or Vocational Technical Education.

Your Alumni Organization

On completion of your program of practical nursing in your respective school, you should want to join your alumni organization. This will give you a feeling of being united with your classmates and other graduates from your school. By attending alumni meetings you will keep up with the progress that your school is making. Often you can help to better the educational program of your school through constructive suggestions. It also gives you an opportunity to familiarize yourself with new developments that are taking place in a hospital as related by an alumnus working in that particular institution. Because membership means "belonging," you have the obligation to be an active member if you join your alumni organization. Plans for continuing education programs are often provided through alumni activities. Projects may be established to provide funds for scholarships to be used by future students in your school. Your alumni organization seeks to encourage the present students to achieve their goals. This may be in the form of an annual tea for the students, a banquet, or a program of entertainment for the students and their parents. Annual dues may be used to enroll annual officers in the national practical nursing organizations or to meet the ever constant need for educational equipment for your school. Your school provided you with the type of education you were seeking; now you should be willing to help other needy students in the school as well as the school itself.

◆ Health and Welfare Insurance, Organizations, and Agencies

Health Insurance

There are many types of insurance available in the United States to protect individuals from some of the financial costs of accident and illness.

Medicare, the health insurance plan under the Social Security Act, went into effect July 1, 1966. Under this plan basic hospital benefits and voluntary supplementary medical insurance were made available for 19 million citizens 65 years of age and older. Since 1966 new Social Security legislation has been enacted, and the benefits of the program have expanded. Some states offer other programs in conjunction with the federal government to help defray medical expenses for low income residents or welfare assistance recipients. This program is known as Medicaid; different states vary in eligibility and requirements.

Medicare includes two parts. Part A is the hospital insurance and is financed by special contributions from employers, employees, and self-employed persons. Part B is the medical insurance; it is financed jointly by the federal government and by the basic medical insurance policies of those who enroll voluntarily when they become 65 years of age.

Part A (hospital insurance) helps to pay some hospitalization costs and contributes to related health services that may be required when the patient leaves the hospital. The hospital benefits are limited to certain maximum amounts for specified periods of time. The "benefit period" can begin again if the person has not received skilled nursing care for 60 consecutive days. Some benefits included are as follows:

1. Inpatient hospital benefits include semiprivate rooms with regular nursing care; meals, including special diets; operating room charges, including recovery room charges; intensive care nursing; medical supplies such as traction, braces, crutches, and walkers; social services; drugs; laboratory tests; and x-ray examinations and other radiology services.
2. Extended care benefits after leaving the hospital, provided the physician

determines the patient needs such care, are the same as the hospital benefits shown previously. The physician must order care in an extended care facility (ECF) at least 3 days after hospitalization or within 14 days after the patient has left the hospital.

3. Home health benefits are available when the physician decides that continued care is needed in the patient's home by a home health agency following the patient's discharge from a hospital or ECF. These benefits include social services; speech, occupational, and physical therapy; part-time nursing and home health aide care; and the use of medical supplies and medical appliances.

Part B (medical insurance) helps to pay for some of the patient's covered medical expenses when they exceed the specified amount that is deductible each year. Some benefits included are as follows:

1. Physician's service in the office, in the outpatient department, at home, or in the hospital
2. Drugs that must be administered by the physician and cannot be self-administered
3. Hospital outpatient services, including diagnosis and treatment (special limitations on psychiatric care)
4. Specified services of a podiatrist
5. Miscellaneous health and medical services ordered by a physician, such as diagnostic services; x-ray and radiation treatments; physical therapy; surgical dressings, casts, and braces; and rental of equipment such as a hospital bed, walker, or other equipment to be used in the home

Of the approximately 2000 private insurance agencies, Blue Cross is the largest single supplier of hospital insurance. Its plans usually cover the hospital room, regular nursing care, laboratory services, x-ray examinations, electrocardiograms, drugs, dressings, special treatments, operating and delivery rooms, and many other hospital services. Membership must be transferred when members move to another area. Hospitalization insurance should be included in the family budget because hospital care is a part of life.

There are various types of insurance plans designed to help meet the costs of sickness and accidents. Blue Cross and Blue Shield policies are generally accepted as the main plans in many areas of the country. Many plans encourage the use of preventive care (health maintenance organizations) and will cover medical costs for the insured even when there is no hospitalization. You should know and understand the policy before you take it because the benefits, including length of time covered, surgery, medical expenses, and nursing care, may vary greatly with each policy.

For several years now much has been said about the need for an effective form of national health insurance to benefit all citizens. Several plans have been proposed, but there seems to be no real agreement at this time as to which kind of plan is needed.

Some type of plan that will offer unlimited possibilities for new kinds of health care undoubtedly will be developed within the coming years. Be sure to follow political developments and proposals closely through nursing journals and other sources. It is very possible that you, the practical nurse, will be involved in the planning stages of preventive care and health education.

Health Maintenance Organization (HMO)

An HMO is a prepaid highly organized system of health care. The concept of the HMO is aimed at preventing illness and maintaining health through routine health examinations, close observation, early diagnosis of disease, and health teaching. Members of an HMO pay a monthly or quarterly membership fee and for this receive standard, essential health services.

The prevention of disease is a medically and economically sound philosophy. It costs less to keep persons healthy than to cure them once they are ill. A diagnostic office visit is cheaper than a stay in the hospital.

Once a client becomes a member of an HMO he is entitled to all the services. He must choose as his primary physician one of the HMO's staff. Physicians employed by the HMO receive a salary, and this salary is not based on the number of patients he sees. A member's fee, too, remains the same whether he sees a physician once a year or once a week. All basic health services are rendered at a central location. Some large HMOs have their own hospitals; however, most have contracts with hospitals that provide many varied and diagnostic services.

Nurses are an important part of an HMO. They function as primary health practitioners, working with physicians, not for physicians.

Government Health and Welfare Organizations

To provide better care for the patient in the community and to promote health and the prevention of illness, hospitals are now working closely with many health and welfare organizations outside the hospital.

Department of Health and Human Services (DHHS). The DHHS, established in 1953 as the Department of Health, Education, and Welfare, helps promote the general welfare of the entire population. It has been reorganized several times to better meet its many responsibilities. To carry out fully its programs in health, welfare, vocational rehabilitation, consumer protection, and social security, Title VI of the Civil Rights Act of 1964 prohibiting discrimination needed to be enforced. Major reorganizations again occurred in 1966 after the creation of a new administration on aging. The largest amount of money is used by nonfederal agencies, institutions, and individuals necessitating various partnerships for the improvement of our society.

DDHS is a cabinet level department, with the Secretary advising the President on programs of the Federal government pertaining to welfare, health, and income security plans. The DHHS is concerned with people of all ages, from newborn infants to the elderly, by mailing out social security checks and making health services more widely available.

Office of Human Development Services (OHDS). The OHDS is responsible for administering programs designed to deal with specific population problems, such as children of low income families, handicapped persons, runaway youth, the elderly, American Indians, native Alaskans, and native Hawaiians.

Social Security Administration. The Social Security Administration was established in 1935 by the United States government. As the needs of the people changed, the basic program has been changed. This national health program includes old age, survivors', and disability insurance, which now covers almost all persons who are employed.

Most working people in the United States are now establishing protection for themselves and their families by paying their Social Security contributions. During working years employees, their employers, and self-employed people pay social security contributions into a special trust fund. When a worker retires, becomes disabled, or dies, benefits in the form of monthly checks are paid to individuals or families to replace part of the earnings lost. Part of the contributions go into a hospital trust fund that is used to help pay hospital bills when workers and their dependents reach 65. Because changes occur very rapidly, contact the Social Security office nearest you for current information.

Administered by each state, social insurance against other risks is provided through workmen's compensation and unemployment insurance. In addition to these social insurance programs, there is a program of federal grants to the states to help them provide financial assistance, medical care, and other services for each state's needy people.

Social Security cards. Nursing is covered by the Social Security Act; thus you must have a Social Security number. This number, which is shown on your Social Security card, is used to keep a record of your earnings. You should use the same number all your life. Both your name and number are needed to make sure that you get credit for your earnings. You should show your card to each employer so that your name and number will be used to report your wages correctly. If you are self-employed, copy your name and number exactly as they appear on the card on the form you use to report your net earnings for Social Security credit.

If there is a Social Security office in your town, it will help you get a Social Security card or get a duplicate card to replace one if it is lost or if you change your name. Be sure the new card shows the same number. If there is no Social Security office in your town, you may obtain an application blank from your post office.

The law requires each employer to give you a receipt for the Social Security taxes that have been deducted from your pay. This is done at the end of each year and when you terminate employment. These receipts (W-2 forms) will help you check on your Social Security because they show the amount deducted as well as the wages paid you. You may check the total earnings reported for you by obtaining an addressed postcard from your Social Security office, signing it, and sending it back, or you may write the Social Security Administration, Baltimore, MD 21235, and request a statement of your account. This statement will show the amount of earnings reported for you. It does not show the amount of taxes paid. Benefits are based on earnings, not on the amount of taxes paid.

Public Health Service. The Public Health Service (Room 17-22, 5600 Fishers Lane, Rockville, MD 20852), created by an act in 1789, has been broadened to cover the responsibility of improving and protecting the environment and health of the people of the nation. These services also work in cooperation with other countries and international organizations involved in world health planning. Since 1967 the Public Health Service has been divided into six major agencies: Food and Drug Administration; the National Institutes of Health; Alcohol, Drug Abuse, and Mental Health Administration; Centers for Disease Control; Health Services Administration; and Health Administration.

Food and Drug Administration. The Food and Drug Administration (HFI-10, 5600 Fishers Lane, Rockville, MD 20852) was established in 1906 and has been known under several organizational titles. It is made up of several Bureaus whose main functions are to protect the health of the nation against potential hazards, impure and unsafe drugs, foods, and cosmetics. Some examples are (1) research programs conducted to study biological effects and long-term exposure to potentially toxic chemicals; (2) policies on labeling all drugs, evaluation of new drugs, quality of drugs, and effectiveness of over-the-counter drugs; and (3) standards set up after research on food for quality, safety, food additives, nutrition, and cosmetics.

The National Institutes of Health. The National Institutes of Health (Building #1, Room 307, Bethesda, MD 20014) was established to improve the American people's health. This is accomplished by conducting research into the causes, prevention, and cure of disease; development and support of research training and services; and communicating biological and medical information using current methods.

This organization is made up of several institutes and divisions for specific subjects, such as the National Institute on Aging.

Alcohol, Drug Abuse, and Mental Health Administration (ADAMHA). The ADAMHA (Room 16-95, 5600 Fishers Lane, Rockville, MD 20852) was established at the federal level to provide leadership in the reduction and elimination of alcohol and drug abuse health problems. This organization is responsible for prevention, control, treatment, and rehabilitation of persons affected by alcohol abuse, drug abuse, and mental illness.

Health Services Administration (HSA). The HSA (Room 14A-55, 5600 Fishers Lane, Rockville, MD 20852) was established to provide leadership in the delivery of health services. Through bureaus, health care services are provided for migrant workers, maternal and child welfare, family planning, community health, Indian health, Federal beneficiaries and native Alaskans. These services are provided through hospitals, clinics, and ambulatory health care centers in urban and rural areas.

State health departments. State health departments are supported by state funds and are under the jurisdiction of the governors of the states, who appoint various officials responsible for the local departments. The departments and officials included vary from state to state. Some state health departments are responsible for the licensing of nursing homes, hospitals, undertakers, beauticians, and manufacturers, as well as providing film libraries, assistance to the local departments, and educational materials (usually free). Other state divisions work in the areas of mental health, nutrition, venereal disease, vital statistics, communicable disease control, public health nursing, laboratories, research, sanitation, and maternal and child health.

Local health departments. Local health departments have many of the same duties as the state health departments; however, the functions differ with each county, city, or township, depending on available funds and their use. The quality and quantity of services given are affected at the local level by the mayor, county supervisor, councilmen, county managers, and commissioners. Their routine responsibilities ordinarily include (1) reporting all communicable diseases; (2) maternal and child health, dental health, nutrition, mental health, and schools; (3) vital statistics, accurate record keeping of birth, death, population, disease, marriage, and divorce rates; (4) environmental sanitation; and (5) public health nursing and health education.

World Health Organization (WHO). The main function of WHO is to assist countries in strengthening their own health services through the advice of public health experts in disease control. Other functions include international sanitary regulations, uniform registration of diseases and deaths, standardization of important drugs, and control of communicable diseases throughout the world.

Food stamp program. The food stamp program was initiated in 1961 by the Department of Agriculture as a method of helping low income and welfare-aided families to buy needed food. The federal government makes up the difference between the amount the family pays and the total value of the coupons. The coupons may be used to buy all foods, excluding those imported.

Private and Voluntary Health Agencies

Private and voluntary health agencies receive funds through donations, gifts, United Way, membership fees, and sometimes public funds. Public funds may be given to a voluntary hospital as payment for some service that is considered a public responsibility, such as for an indigent patient.

Because of difficulties incurred through administration at a national level, most private agencies are operated on a state or local level. If you have no agency in your area to meet a specific need and help is needed for your patient, you may write to the National Health Council, 1740 Broadway, New York, NY 10019, for the location of the nearest state or local office.

Some of these private and voluntary agencies are as follows:

1. Alcoholics Anonymous—helps any alcoholic who desires help. Alcoholics Anonymous groups throughout the world are made up of recovered alcoholics. They share their recovery to help other alcoholics overcome their problem.
2. American Cancer Society—constitutes a threefold program of research, education, and service aimed at controlling and eliminating cancer. It provides service and rehabilitation counseling, transportation, and loan-closet items (sickroom supplies and comfort items). Volunteers assist in rehabilitation of

laryngectomy, mastectomy, and ostomy patients. Other patient assistance programs, specific to each local division, are also available.

3. American Diabetes Association—provides education to the public and to professionals regarding the nature and treatment of diabetes. It distributes accurate information to the public and to patients. It improves standards of treatment and promotes research.

4. American Heart Association, Inc.—provides educational programs for professionals, patients, and the general public. It supports research and sets standards to maintain better medical care for patients with cardiovascular diseases.

5. American National Red Cross—chosen by the Congress to help carry out the obligations assumed by the United States under certain international treaties known as the Geneva or Red Cross Conventions. A volunteer 50-member Board of Governors directs the activities of the Red Cross, which are carried out by the managers of four national field offices through 70 divisions and 3142 local chapters. The Congressional charter imposes on the American Red Cross two of its programs: services to the armed forces, veterans, and their families and disaster services. Other programs, all of which are designed to meet human needs, are the blood program, community health and safety programs (first aid, small craft, water safety, and nursing and health), youth service programs, community volunteer programs, and international services.

6. Arthritis and Rheumatism Foundation—conducts research, promotes educational programs, supports treatment facilities, and assists in physician and other health care personnel training in prevention, diagnosis, and treatment of arthritis.

7. Association for the Aid of Crippled Children (and adults)—offers instructional materials, conducts research and scientific conferences for health care providers, and prepares educational literature for patients. This organization receives some funds from Easter Seals.

8. Muscular Dystrophy Association of America, Inc.—conducts research for the discovery of a cause and cure for muscular dystrophy. It assists in the purchase and repair of appliances and provides physical therapy, transportation, education, and counseling.

9. National Society for the Prevention of Blindness—cooperates with local organizations such as parents' groups, fraternal organizations, health-related institutions, and governmental agencies in sight conservation programs. It gives vision-screening tests and publishes a wide variety of educational and teaching materials. It offers industry safety incentive programs and awards research grants in a wide variety of areas with potential application to prevention of blindness.

10. National Association for Mental Health—conducts clinical research, provides educational programs, and works for improved preventative and treatment facilities. It informs the public about ways to avoid mental breakdown.

11. National Coordinating Council of Drug Abuse—evaluates educational programs, assists in research, and sets up interdisciplinary committees by area needs. It coordinates educational and informational efforts of groups on drug abuse.
12. National Multiple Sclerosis Society—offers a research program in finding the cause, treatment, and cure of this disease. It provides educational literature for health care providers, victims, and the public.
13. Planned Parenthood—conducts research, makes educational literature available, and deals with issues of family size, child spacing, marriage, infertility, and family stability.
14. Visiting Nurses' Association—provides nursing at home under a physician's orders for the acutely ill, chronically ill, invalids, mothers and newborn babies, convalescents, and others who are unable to leave home for treatment. This agency teaches members of the family to give patient care, as well as assisting the patient in regaining and maintaining health.

In addition to the organizations just listed, there are many programs administered at the local level.

◆ Home Care Related Organizations

The following is a partial list of the national groups and associations that may help the home caregiver.

Aging
American Association of Retired Persons (AARP)
    1909 K St., N.W.
    Washington, DC 20049
    (202) 872-4700
The National Association of Area Agencies on Aging (N4A)
    600 Maryland Ave., S.W.
    Suite 208-W
    Washington, DC 20024
    (202) 484-7520
National Support Center for Families of the Aging
    P.O. Box 245
    Swarthmore, PA 19081

Home Care
Foundation for Hospice and Homecare
    519 C St., N.E.
    Stanton Park
    Washington, DC 20002
    (202) 547-6586

National Association for Home Care
    519 C St., N.E.
    Stanton Park
    Washington, DC 20002
    (202) 547-7424

Self-Help Clearing Houses
The National Self Help Clearinghouse
    c/o City University of New York
    33 W. 42nd St.
    New York, NY 10036
    (212) 840-1259
The Self Help Center
    1600 Dodge Ave.
    Suite S-122
    Evanston, IL 60201
    (312) 328-0470

◆ *Study Helps*

1. List two journals published especially for the practical nurse and give the publisher of each.
2. Explain NAPNES and state its functions.
3. Explain NFLPN and state its functions.
4. Explain NLN and state its functions.
5. Explain ANA and state its functions.
6. What is the purpose of an alumni organization? What is your obligation toward it?
7. List six health and welfare organizations and state their functions.

Bibliography

Cornacchia HJ and Barrett S: Consumer health: a guide to intelligent decisions, ed 2, St Louis, 1980, The CV Mosby Co.

De Young L: Dynamics of nursing, ed 5, St Louis, 1984, The CV Mosby Co.

Reinhardt AM and Quinn MD: Family-centered community nursing, St Louis, 1980, The CV Mosby Co.

Saxton DF, Nugent PM, and Pelikan P: Mosby's comprehensive review of nursing, ed 12, St Louis, 1987, The CV Mosby Co.

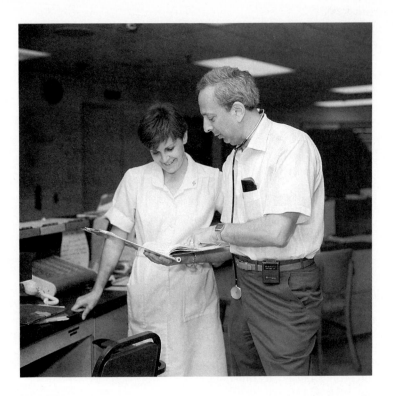

Objectives

At the completion of this chapter the student practical nurse will be able to:

◆ Discuss the supervisory role of the practical nurse.

◆ Explain basic principles of group dynamics.

◆ List practical supervisory techniques that can be used in the clinical area.

◆ Identify personal values.

◆ Explain the role of communications in supervision.

Leadership and the Practical Nurse

Gloria E. Wold

◆ The Need for Leadership Skills

Because of today's nursing staff shortage in the United States, the health care delivery system requires that each person work to the maximum potential. With the shortage of nurses and the increasing demand for health care by society, the LPN is called on to perform many functions and accept multiple responsibilities. This is particularly true in long-term and extended care facilities. Although each state has different laws and agency policies, the practical nurse is increasingly likely to supervise other employees. Frequently they are expected to function as the charge nurse or team leader. They are expected to supervise aides and nursing assistants and coordinate the day-to-day activities of a ward, unit, or wing.

Frequently an LPN is new to an institution when she is assigned "charge" responsibilities. Not only is she expected to perform skilled nursing care (observational changes, medications, and treatments) for a large number of patients, but she is also expected to supervise and coordinate the work of other less-skilled personnel. This is a great deal of responsibility to assume in a short period. These expectations are unreasonable, but unfortunately this occurs frequently. This amount of responsibility, assumed too quickly, often causes the practical nurse to become frustrated; feeling lost and frustrated she tries to do the best she can. The training has not prepared her for the added responsibilities.

Because of limited time, many nursing schools focus on the clinical nursing skills. Leadership and supervision skills often are not addressed. This gap in nursing education is understandable; technical nursing knowledge has expanded so quickly that there is not enough time to teach everything. However, this is unfortunate, because without quality leadership and supervision, patient care suffers. Some students are fortunate; they seem to be born leaders and adapt easily to the supervisory role. These are the fortunate few. Most students learn leadership skills over a period of time by trial and error. It is hoped that this material will make the transition easier for you.

◆ Legal Implications

Before you accept the responsibilities of team leader or charge nurse you must be aware of the *allowable scope of practice* for a practical nurse in your state. In most states the practical nurse works under the direction of an RN, physician, or other approved medical personnel. This scope is interpreted differently in each state, and sometimes even in different areas of the same state. No textbook can address all of the variations adequately. It is important that you discuss this topic in class so you have a clear understanding of the laws in your state. It is imperative that you do not exceed your legal limitations. Ignorance of the law will not protect you. When dealing with organizational or supervisory problems, or situations in which complex judgments must be made, be sure to seek guidance from your manager. This is similar to what you have learned to do in patient care situations. When a nursing situation regarding a patient becomes too complex or exceeds your level of practice, notify the RN or physician.

When supervising others the same principle is true. When a situation exceeds your scope of practice you must seek guidance. You should not be expected to deal with these situations on your own.

◆ Management and Supervision

Management refers to the highest levels of the organization and is also used to describe the activity of directing the actions of a large number of people. High-level managers or administrators are responsible for making an organization or business succeed. They have a great deal of authority and responsibility. The higher they are in the organizational structure, the greater their responsibility and authority. Some tasks involved in management include planning, preparation of budgets, hiring, firing, and supervising employees. In general they look at the "big picture" concerns of the institution.

Supervision involves directing and inspecting the day-to-day work performance of others. Supervisors usually are in the middle levels of the organization. They have various levels of authority, depending on the institution. Usually they work under the direction of a manager. Supervisors have the responsibility to see that selected tasks are completed either by themselves or by the people they supervise.

◆ Leadership and Supervision

Leadership and supervision are often defined as accomplishing tasks through people. No one person can do everything. Getting things done frequently requires a group effort. To be a good leader and supervisor it is important to understand more about groups and group dynamics.

Groups and Group Dynamics

A group is any number of people who have a common goal. Groups can be large or small, simple or complex, formal or informal. Some examples are businesses, hospitals, families, churches, work teams, clubs, or study groups. Large groups often have several smaller groups within them. Groups take on personalities of their own. Groups have values, and they establish rules to guide the behavior of members.

Organizations such as businesses or hospitals have written goals because of their size and complexity. These are called the philosophy, mission statement, or strategic plan of the organization. Managers have developed a formal organizational structure to regulate and govern the organization. Fig. 4 shows how the individuals and groups within the organization relate to each other. In most situations a hierarchy is formed. This hierarchy illustrates how information moves. The figure also shows the flow of power or authority. The organization sets up rules that outline acceptable behaviors and also defines the rewards and punishments for appropriate and inappropriate behaviors. These rules are found in policy and procedure manuals.

Each person in a formal group is assigned a role. In an organization this becomes a job description, which includes a list of duties and responsibilities. Because of the large number of people, the fixed structure, and the rules, it takes a long time to make decisions and changes in large organizations.

The structure and dynamics of smaller, less formal groups such as families, work groups, or friends who study together are not as easily described. Informal groups have unwritten goals and values. They accept or reject certain behaviors from their members. Each informal group is unique. The members know the rules in their own group. They know how information moves through the group and who the leader is, but an outsider is usually not aware of how each informal group works.

Within informal groups the same person may have several different roles. Decisions and changes are made quickly to respond to the needs of the group. Good observation and communication skills are required if an outsider wants to determine the values, flow of information, and power structure of an informal group.

Conflict

Every person is a member of many different groups. Think for a moment. Try to identify all of the different groups to which you belong. There are groups at home, at school, at work, and in the community. Within one area such as work, each individual may belong to several different formal and informal groups. For example, one person may be a member of the LPN group, the charge nurse/supervisor group, the night shift, the 3-West team, and a member of the infection control committee.

When the goals and values of the formal and informal groups are in harmony and support each other, activities usually go smoothly. Large amounts of work can be accomplished, and people are happy and satisfied while doing the work.

Problems arise when the goals and values of two groups differ significantly, or when one group does not understand the viewpoint of another group. When there is a great deal of difference in values or goals between groups, misunderstandings and conflicts occur. These are manifested as anger, hostility, and resistance, which result in even less communication between the groups. The people involved are unhappy and dissatisfied. Work performance and productivity levels are low. In a health care setting this affects the patients, who become the innocent victims.

Internal conflict and stress can occur when a person has divided loyalty between

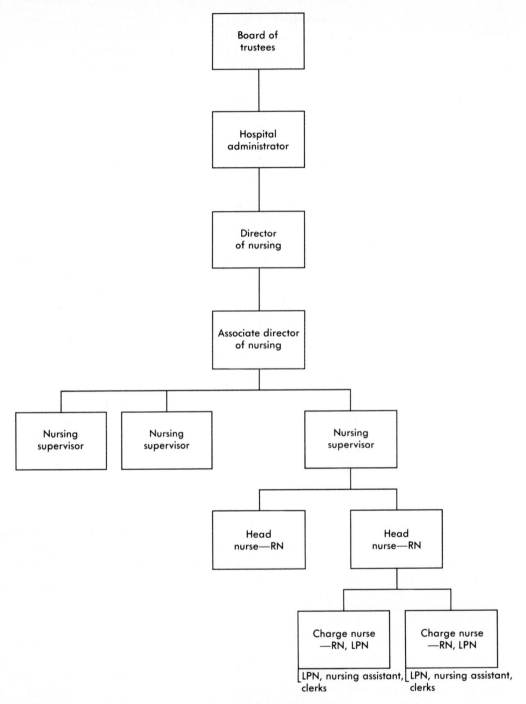

Fig. 4

several groups. If the groups have different goals and values, individuals feel that they are being pulled in different directions by each group. They are not sure which goals or values are right. They often try to please everyone and yet feel that they are not pleasing anyone. Frustration, guilt, and loss of effectiveness, and sometimes even physical symptoms such as headaches result.

You can probably list many conflict situations from personal experience. Simply identifying problems does not help when you are the person in charge. You need to know how to respond. A leader or supervisor can respond to conflict in one of three ways:

1. Become involved in the conflict and make the situation worse.
2. Ignore the conflict and hope it goes away.
3. Take constructive action to prevent or reduce the conflict.

You may ask why anyone would want to make the situation worse. Most leaders do not do this deliberately. They do it by default, usually because of inadequate supervisory skills. Avoidance (trying to ignore conflicts or problems) usually results from the same sense of inadequacy or fear. The only positive choice they can make is to learn better techniques to deal with conflicts and problems. These are called the *basic supervisory skills*.

Values Clarification

Before you attempt to lead or supervise others it is essential that you know yourself. Your values will, to a large extent, determine your attitudes and actions. Your strengths and weaknesses should also be identified. In supervision you should always try to work with your strengths and away from your weaknesses. Unfortunately, most people have not clearly identified these strengths and weaknesses.

If you have never taken time to look seriously at yourself, do so now. Take time to do the exercises at the end of the chapter and see what they reveal about you. This may help you understand yourself better.

◆ Communication Skills

Communication skills are essential to all phases of life. You have learned about communication from the first day you entered nursing school. An earlier chapter of this text gives a good review of some basic principles. The relationship of communication to supervision has been referred to as one and the same thing. An effective supervisor is an effective communicator. Review the following skills and apply them to supervision.

Listening

Listening to others is the most difficult communication skill to acquire. Many things get in the way of effective listening. Hearing is not listening. Listening requires close attention and concentration. Ineffective listening can result in confusion, wasted time, poor morale and is potentially harmful to patients. For example, while caring for a patient you observe a change in vital signs. You report this to the team leader who is passing medications. You think it is important that she has this information promptly, because the physician is due on the unit shortly. She "listens" to you, but 15 minutes later when the physician arrives she calls you away from your duties to get the current vital signs for the same patient. Remember, it is easy to see this behavior in someone else, but difficult to see in ourselves. A short quiz on listening skills at the end of the chapter will give you an idea of how good a listener you are.

The following list identifies some common listening blocks to communication and offers more effective actions that the supervisor can take.

Listening Blocks	Effective Listening Techniques
Too busy with something else	Focus on the message. If you are too busy, explain this and schedule a time when you can give your full attention. Write down information when it is given to you.
Too busy thinking about reply to listen	Focus on what the speaker is saying, not on what you are thinking.
Not interested in the message or pretends to listen	Recognize that as the supervisor you should be interested in your staff and all aspects of patient care.
Too many distractions	Find a quiet place to talk away from the nurses' station and telephone.
Thinks she already knows what the message is	Verify the information. Ask questions until you are sure you have the correct facts.

Although listening is a large part of communication, sending messages appropriately is also an important skill for the supervisor.

Verbal Communications

In supervision you are called on to give directions and information to your staff. You are the bridge between the policies of the formal organization and the day-to-day work. You must deliver messages, coordinate activities, and give specific information regarding the patients and the tasks that need to be done. Suggestions for improved verbal communication are:

Schedule a report meeting at the beginning of the shift. The nursing assistants need to know any changes in patient status or care before they start the day's activities.

Hold the meeting away from distractions. A special meeting room is recommended.

Describe work assignments clearly.

Focus on the information the assistant needs to know.

Keep your directions simple and avoid using abbreviations.

Have nursing assistants briefly repeat any unusual directions to be certain that they understand.

Give your assistants time to ask any questions and clarify your directions.

Keep your staff informed. Get information to people quickly. If anything changes let your staff know immediately.

Written Communication

There are times when a written message is more appropriate than a verbal one. Written messages are tangible. They can be referred to whenever needed. If you do not want instructions to be forgotten or missed, write them down.

As a supervisor you may be expected to communicate in writing to other departments in the facility. These are some times you want to be sure to put things in writing:

Any time a record of the message may be needed at a later time. For example, when making out assignments it is best to back them up in writing so there is no confusion about responsibilities.

When much of the material is new to the worker. New employees may require more written information on the assignment sheet.

If the message is complicated or has several steps.

When the message will be sent to someone in another area or on another shift.

When the same message will go to several different people.

When you do use the written method of communication be sure that your thoughts are clearly written. Use correct grammar and punctuation, and make sure that your writing is legible.

Nonverbal Communication

You can talk about the need to give quality care and respond to patients promptly, but are you a good role model? If a signal light goes on do you answer it, or do you excuse yourself because you are busy with something else? As the charge nurse you have many responsibilities that you cannot delegate to your assistants, but if they are busy and you have time, help them. Let your actions show cooperation and team spirit. Demonstrate the types of response and interaction you want them to have with patients. If you want to receive courteous treatment, then you must treat others, including your staff, courteously.

Rapport and Empathy

You have studied empathy and rapport as they relate to patients. The same skills apply to supervision. It is important that you recognize the importance of the people who work under your direction. Some guidelines to help with this are:

Always try to understand the other person's point of view.

Develop a climate of mutual respect.

Do not let your authority go to your head.

Never put your staff members down.

Keep relationships friendly and productive.

Give encouragement and recognize each person's unique strengths.

◆ Motivation

Nursing is hard work. There are few professions that demand so much from a person with so few tangible rewards. People who provide for the day-to-day needs of patients usually do so for reasons other than financial gain. They feel that they are needed, that what they do is important, and that they do make a difference. As a supervisor you must whenever possible reward the positive behaviors and actions of your staff. By word and action you should demonstrate that they are important. Some ways of doing this are:

Set attainable work loads and standards.

Be fair and equitable in assignments.

Ask for suggestions on how to improve the work atmosphere.

Give praise when it is deserved.

Compliment people on what they did right.

Celebrate small things.

◆ Time Management and Organization

You can have the most highly motivated group working for you, but if they are not organized things will not get done the way they should. As supervisor you are responsible for seeing that the assigned work gets done, and that it gets done on time.

Because we cannot manage time, we need to learn to manage ourselves. Everyone has the same number of hours in a day, yet some people accomplish much more than others. Here are some key ideas for getting things done effectively and efficiently.

Start each day with a written overview of what needs to be done:

How many patients do you have?

What are their needs?

What assessments, medications, and treatments are needed?

Which patients have appointments? When and where?

Are there physician rounds?

Prioritize your activities:

Do the most important things first.

Identify those activities that *must* be done at a specified time and plan ahead for them.

Identify those things that you must do yourself.

Assign routine activities to your staff.

Plan ahead:

Gather all necessary supplies, but make sure that you leave adequate supplies for the next shift.

Plan your steps:

Concentrate on one thing at a time.

Plan your stops in a logical order.

Write things down:

Carry a notebook or worksheet to note things immediately so you do not forget.

Identify the departments you deal with most often such as Pharmacy and Central Processing and Dispatch.

List all questions for these departments together so you can settle everything at one time.

Making Assignments

Part of good organization is proper utilization of your nursing assistants. Listed here are some suggestions:

Make sure that the assigned duties do not exceed the legal limitations or institutional policies.

Consider the strengths and skills of each individual. Match these with the patient's needs.

Provide continuity of care whenever possible.

Consider the physical layout of your unit. Save time by clustering assignments whenever possible.

Do not play favorites. Keep work assignments as fair as possible.

Try various staffing techniques. Use pairs or teams to cover groups of patients.

Problem Employees

It is hoped that most of your staff will be dependable and conscientious. In some cases you may have to work with people who manifest undesirable behaviors. As soon as you are aware of problems, report them to the RN manager and keep her informed. These are some things that you can do to alleviate problems:

Document the facts, not your perceptions. Report in writing to your supervisor the facts and be specific.

Make sure the individual knows what behavior is expected. Verify that directions are understood, and determine whether the person needs more training or assistance.

If you must give corrections do so in private. Do not criticize or reprimand in public.

Stay calm; do not lose your temper.

◆ Values Clarification Exercises

For each exercise number a sheet of paper from 1 to 10, or use 10 slips of paper. Write the first 10 thoughts or statements that come to mind. Do not judge the ideas as you write them down. After you have written 10 different replies to each exercise go back and rank them in order going from that which best describes you or is most important (rank this as number 1) and continue to that which least describes you or is least important (rank this number 10).

Exercise 1

Who am I?   **Importance**

1. _____   _____

2. _____   _____

3. _____   _____

4. _____   _____

5. _____   _____

6. _____   _____

7. _____   _____

8. _____   _____

9. _____   _____

10. _____   _____

(Set up the same as above for remaining exercises.)

Exercise 2   **Things I like to do**

Exercise 3   **People with whom I like to spend time**

Exercise 4   **Things I like about myself**

Exercise 5   **Things I would like to improve**

Exercise 6   **When I am angry I . . .**

Exercise 7   **When someone is supervising me I want them to . . .**

◆ **Listening Skills Quiz**

Directions: Read the following questions, then rate yourself accordingly.

4 points if always
3 points if almost always
2 points if rarely
1 point if never

_____   1. Do I allow the speaker to finish a complete thought before asking questions or interrupting?

_____   2. Do I listen between the lines and look for nonverbal cues or hidden meanings?

_____   3. Do I listen without becoming upset if the speaker's point of view is different from my own?

_____   4. Do I write down important facts or information so I will not forget?

_____   5. If I am interrupted do I stop and give my total attention to the speaker?

_____   6. If I have been given complicated directions, do I repeat them to the speaker for verification before ending the conversation?

_____   7. Do I listen carefully even if I think the speaker is less intelligent or less experienced than I am?

_____   8. Do I avoid becoming distracted when someone is speaking to me?

_____   9. I try to understand and empathize with the speaker.

_____ 10. I ask questions if I am not sure I understood what the speaker said.

Scoring: If you score above 32 you have excellent listening skills. If your score is 27 to 31 you are an above-average listener. If your score is 22 to 26 you need to practice listening skills, and if your score is 21 or less you need to work on your listening skills. Look at the areas marked rarely or never. These are good places to start making changes.

◆ *Study Helps*

1. List two tasks performed by high level managers.
2. What is involved in supervision?
3. Define leadership and supervision.
4. Define a group.
5. List some of your strengths and weaknesses.
6. Describe how the licensed practical nurse can effectively listen to ancillary personnel.
7. List three reasons you would use written communication.
8. List four ways you can motivate your staff.
9. List three ways you can more effectively manage time.
10. List three styles of leadership and briefly describe each.

Bibliography

Abruzzese RS et al: Practices, ed 1, Springhouse, Pa, 1984, Springhouse Book Co.

Cribbin JJ: Leadership, ed 1, New York, 1981, AMACOM Book Division.

Ellis JR and Nowlis EA: Nursing a human needs approach, ed 4, Boston, 1989, Houghton-Mifflin Co.

Haimann T and Hilgert RL: Supervision: concepts and practices of management, ed 4, Cincinnati, 1987, South-Western Publishing Co.

Moloney MM: Leadership in nursing, ed 1, St Louis, 1979, The CV Mosby Co.

Steele SM and Harmon VM: Values clarification in nursing, ed 2, Norwalk, Conn, 1983, Appleton-Century-Crofts.

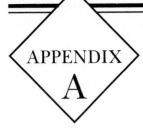

APPENDIX A

Desirable Characteristics for a Leader

1. Listens and is approachable
2. Communicates clearly both verbally and in writing
3. Sets high standards; is honest and trustworthy
4. Is fair and objective
5. Is a doer and sets a positive example
6. Uses positive motivation techniques
7. Is goal directed and organized
8. Shows enthusiasm and a sense of humor
9. Is tactful, humble, and understanding
10. Is knowledgeable and has good judgment

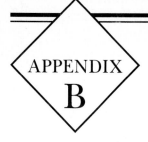

APPENDIX B

Styles of Leadership

Those of you with work experience have probably seen several leadership styles in action. Those of you who have not held jobs can think of teachers or head nurses in clinical agencies that you visited during school.

None of the styles discussed here are right or wrong. The most effective leaders frequently use more than one style. The art of leadership is knowing which style to use at a given time. Much can be learned by observing people in leadership roles and comparing them to the descriptions given below.

◆ Authoritarian Leaders

Some individuals feel that because they have authority or power they should "call the shots" on everything. They often tend to be poor communicators and like to "tell" everybody under their direction what, when, and how to do everything. They let you know immediately that they are the boss. The technical name for this style of leadership is the authoritarian or autocratic style. Authoritarian leaders often do not trust others. They frequently believe that people do not want to work and will do anything to get out of working. Because of this distrust they feel a strong need to maintain control. Most people do not like to work for highly authoritarian leaders, because this style does not allow individual employees to contribute or participate actively in work-related decisions. Most people are likely to be afraid of the authoritarian leader because he has a tendency to be highly critical.

Newly appointed supervisors or team leaders frequently act in an authoritarian manner. This happens for several reasons. Some training programs tend to be authoritarian. The student is expected to follow instructions and not question directions. It is natural for students to model their behaviors on familiar ideas, even if they know that they are not the most effective actions.

Fear can also be a factor when adopting the authoritarian style. When a person is uncertain but wishes to appear in control, it is easier to give orders that seem to indicate knowledge and confidence than acknowledge that an assistant may have valuable knowledge to contribute. Frequently student nurses are expected to have the right answer when questioned by the instructor; indications of uncertainty are not acceptable. This thinking carries over into the new situation and makes admission of the need for help awkward.

Lack of trust is another reason new supervisors adopt the authoritarian style. When you begin to supervise, you realize that you are accepting responsibility for the actions of other people. This comes as a shock to many new supervisors. They have often just gained enough confidence to trust themselves. Suddenly they have to make the additional mental shift to trusting others. This is very difficult, particularly for new graduates. Many people feel that if they give orders and exercise a great deal of control, everything will run smoothly.

Poor communication skills can also be a factor in the authoritarian style. A person who has poor communication skills may have to resort to giving orders. They lack many of the techniques that allow them to do anything else.

Do not infer from this discussion that the authoritarian style is without merit. There are times when giving directions or orders is not only proper, it is necessary.

◆ Democratic Style

Another style of leadership that you may have observed is the democratic style. This is also called the collaborative or participative style of leadership. The democratic leader is in charge. He or she is responsible for providing direction to the group. The difference between authoritarian and democratic styles is that the participative leader attempts to include all of the staff in the decision-making process. Group members are actively involved in setting goals; therefore they are usually more committed to seeing that these goals are achieved.

Democratic leaders usually have a different view of people from that of authoritarian leaders. They are more likely to trust people, usually because they have greater confidence themselves. They think that people want to work and desire to do their jobs well. Good understanding of communications and human relations skills is a common trait of democratic leaders. The authoritarian gives orders, whereas the democratic leader guides and directs. In most cases groups working under a democratic leader get more work done and are happier doing the work.

There is also a negative side to the democratic style. Establishing a democratic climate takes time. It takes a group of strangers time to learn to trust the democratic leader. Because this style is not familiar to many people, they may not be sure if the leader really wants their input. It also takes longer to get ideas and information from several people before making a decision than it takes if one person makes the decision.

◆ Laissez-Faire Style

This term comes from the French language. The literal translation is "allow them to do." Another way of saying this is "anything goes." The leader does not interfere but lets the group do as they please. Some individuals who have grown up in a very authoritarian system will go to the opposite extreme and never give orders or directions. This frequently results in chaos, with little work being accomplished. Because there is no direction or guidance in a laissez-faire system, people often are confused and unsure of what is expected of them. This is not an effective style in most settings and in a health care setting it can result in total disaster.

◆ Task-Oriented Style Versus People-Oriented Style

Some supervisors focus on accomplishing tasks. They see a day as a list of jobs to be done. This list of tasks is divided among the staff until everything gets done. Little attention is paid to the people who have to do the work. The workers are viewed as a means to an end. Individual abilities, likes, and dislikes are all secondary to getting the job done. Most nurses tend to be very task-oriented. They frequently see their day as a list of orders, medications, appointments, and treatments. This is an unrealistic perception of the profession. Because of this approach they may lose track of the people (both patients and employees). People-oriented leaders focus more on the individual involved than the tasks. They may know that the tasks are important, but they do not want to hurt anybody's feelings. However, this situation rarely lasts because the tasks are not completed as expected.

The most workable style is a combination of both the task-oriented and people-oriented styles. The ideal is to balance a task- and people-oriented attitude. This combination recognizes that there are many tasks to be done, but that the people involved are important also.

◆ Situational or Eclectic Style

As stated earlier no single style is always appropriate. The most effective leaders select aspects from several styles as the situation requires. The eclectic leader realizes that both the tasks and the people involved are important. In situations involving nursing care the supervising nurse must keep complete control. If something must be done, or must be done in a particular way, it is the leader's responsibility to see that it is done promptly and correctly. Nurses reporting to the supervisor must recognize her authority and responsibility. In cases of emergency the supervisor must know that an order will be followed.

In other areas, however, the nurse in charge may use a more democratic style. Making daily assignments, assigning miscellaneous tasks, and scheduling breaks and lunch are simple examples of where the employees could and should have input. These areas affect the employee directly and can greatly impact job satisfaction.

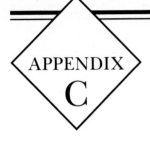

APPENDIX C

Test Plan for the NCLEX-PN and Test-Taking Skills

The NCSBN's test plan for the NCLEX-PN encompasses eight categories of practical/vocational nursing activities. Each category is vital to the assurance of the final intent of the examination: to protect the public through safe practitioners. The eight categories as given in the actual test plan, including the percent of questions allocated to each specific category on the examination, are listed on the following pages.

♦ *Test Plan for the National Council Licensure Examination for Practical Nurses*

I. Communicating and Participating in Plans of Care (3%-7%)
Incorporates participation in the development and evaluation of plans of care as a member of the health care team; providing emotional support and guidance to the patient and significant others; communicating effectively with all concerned; and health teaching within the P/VN scope of practice.

II. Administering Special Therapies: Medications/Oxygen (13%-17%)
Incorporates all those aspects of medication administration, oxygen therapy administration, and monitoring of intravenous therapy relative to the scope of P/VN practice.

III. Providing for Therapeutic Needs (18%-22%)
Incorporates numerous therapeutic and lifesaving procedures within the realm of P/VN activities, such as pre- and postoperative care, nasopharynx suctioning, catheterization, cast care, and cardiopulmonary resuscitation (CPR).

IV. Providing for Basic Health Needs (8%-12%)
Incorporates principles relative to specific therapies and patient needs such as the application of heat and cold, proper body mechanics and alignment, comfort and safety and normal nutrition.

V. Collecting and Recording Information (17%-21%)
Incorporates the measurement and recording of all those aspects pertinent to, for example, signs and symptoms of major health problems; body structure and function; assisting with special examinations; predisposing factors to illness; and the principles, as well as the legal aspects, of charting.

VI. Maintaining Safety (14%-18%)
Incorporates principles of sterile and aseptic technique, as well as all other aspects of patient safety and rights.

VII. Promoting Hygiene and Self-care (10%-14%)
Incorporates principles relative to daily living activities, basic hygiene and orientation of patient to his/her own environment.

VIII. Maintaining a Healthy Environment (1%-5%)
Incorporates a variety of environmental principles necessary for maintaining patient safety and rights, as well as for administering quality nursing care.

Adapted from the National Council of State Boards of Nursing, Inc., Chicago, October 1984.
From Yannes-Eyles M: Mosby's Comprehensive Review of Practical Nursing, ed 10, St Louis, 1990, The CV Mosby Co.

◆ *Test-Taking Skills*

Begin with a positive attitude about yourself, your nursing knowledge, and your test-taking abilities. A positive attitude is achieved through self-confidence gained by studying effectively. One of the keys to taking this exam is to "over-study" throughout the year. Do not try to cram for the test.

Be emotionally prepared for the examination. Get a good night's sleep. In the morning allow yourself plenty of time to dress, have breakfast, and arrive at the testing site a few minutes early. Practicing a few relaxation techniques may also prove helpful to you.

Listen to the examiner and read the written directions carefully. Failure to listen or read the directions thoroughly may result in an incorrect answer, which could cause you considerable loss of points. Should you have any question regarding the directions, ask the examiner for clarification.

Answer *all* questions. You are scored on the number of questions you answer correctly, not on how many you answer wrong. You have at least a 25% chance of selecting the correct answer.

Remember there is a time factor involved, so do not spend an excessive amount of time on any one question. One minute should be the maximum time allotted to any question. If you find it necessary to move on, make a note of the question and return to it later.

Each question contains a stem (the main intent of the question), followed by four plausible answers or alternatives that either complete a statement or answer the question presented. Only one of the alternatives is the *best* answer; the remaining alternatives are known as distractors because they are written in such a way that they could be the correct answer and distract you to a certain degree. Therefore answer each question carefully.

Read, do not scan, the situation and question carefully, looking for key words or phrases.

Key words or phrases in the stem of the question, such as first, primary, early, and best, are important. Likewise, words such as only, always, never, and all in the alternatives will frequently be evidence of a wrong response.

Have confidence in your initial response to a question; it will probably be the correct answer. If you are unable to answer immediately, eliminate the alternatives you know are incorrect and proceed from there. This will increase your chances of randomly selecting the correct answer.

Many times the correct answer is the longest alternative given; however, do not count on it. Individuals who prepare the examination are also aware of this fact and avoid offering you any "helpful hints."

Avoid looking for an answer pattern or code. Many times four or five consecutive questions will have the same letter or number for the correct answer.

Be alert for grammatical inconsistencies. If the response is intended to complete the stem (an incomplete sentence) but makes no grammatical sense to you, it can be considered to be a distractor rather than the correct answer. However, great effort is expended by test developers to eliminate such inconsistencies.

Adapted from Yannes-Eyles, Mosby's Comprehensive Review of Practical Nursing, ed 10, St Louis, 1990, The CV Mosby Co.

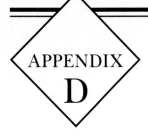

APPENDIX D

State and Territorial Boards of Nursing and Practical Nursing

Alabama

Executive Officer, Alabama Board of Nursing, Suite 203, 500 East Boulevard, Montgomery 36117, (205) 261-4060

Alaska

Executive Officer, Alaska Board of Nursing, (907) 561-2878
For licensing information
Licensing Examiner, Board of Nursing, P.O. Box D-LIC, Dept. of Commerce and Economic Development, Div. of Occupational Licensing, Juneau 99811, (907) 465-2544

Arizona

Executive Secretary, Arizona State Board of Nursing, 2001 W. Camelback, Suite 350, Phoenix 85015, (602) 255-5092

Arkansas

Executive Director, Arkansas State Board of Nursing, University Towers Bldg., Suite 800, 1123 S. University, Little Rock 72204, (501) 371-2751

California

Executive Officer, California Board of Registered Nursing, 1030 13th St., Suite 200, Sacramento 95814, (916) 322-3350

Executive Secretary, California Board of Vocational Nurse and Psychiatric Technical Examiners, 1414 K St., Sacramento 95814, (916) 323-2167

Colorado

Program Administrator, Colorado Board of Nursing, 1560 Broadway, Suite 670, Denver 80202, (303) 894-2430

Connecticut

Executive Secretary, Connecticut Board of Nursing, 150 Washington Street, Hartford 06106, (203) 566-1032

Delaware

Executive Director, Delaware Board of Nursing, Margaret O'Neill Bldg., P.O. Box 1401, Dover 19901, (302) 736-4752

District of Columbia

President, District of Columbia Board of Nursing, 614 H Street, N.W., Washington 20001, (202) 727-7468

Florida

Executive Director, Florida Board of Nursing, 111 Coastline Drive East, Suite 504, Jacksonville 32202, (904) 359-6331

Georgia

Executive Director, Georgia Board of Nursing, 166 Pryor Street, S.W., Atlanta 30303, (404) 656-3921

Executive Director, Georgia State Board of Licensed Practical Nurses, 166 Pryor Street, S.W., Atlanta 30303, (404) 656-3921

For licensing information

Joint Secretary, Georgia State Examining Boards, 166 Pryor Street, S.W., Atlanta 30303, (404) 656-3900

Guam

Nurse Examiner Administrator, Guam Board of Nurse Examiners, Dept. of Public Health & Social Services, P.O. Box 2816, Agana 96901, (671) 734-4813

Hawaii

Executive Secretary, Board of Nursing, State of Hawaii, P.O. Box 3469, Honolulu 96801, (808) 548-3086

Idaho

Executive Director, Idaho Board of Nursing, 500 South 10th St., Suite 102, Boise 83720, (208) 334-3110

Illinois

Assistant Deputy Director, Illinois Department of Professional Regulation/Nursing Section, 320 West Washington Street, Springfield 62786, (217) 782-4386

Indiana

President, Indiana State Board of Nursing, Health Professions Service Bureau, One American Square, Suite 1020, Box 82067, Indianapolis 46282-0004, (317) 232-2960

Iowa

Executive Director, Iowa Board of Nursing, Executive Hills East, 1223 East Court, Des Moines 50319, (515) 281-3256

Kansas

Executive Administrator, Kansas Board of Nursing, Landon State Office Bldg., 900 S.W. Jackson, Suite 551-S, Topeka 66612, (913) 296-4929

Kentucky

Executive Director, Kentucky State Board of Nursing, 4010 Dupont Circle, Suite 430, Louisville 40207, (502) 897-5143

Louisiana

Executive Director, Louisiana State Board of Nursing, 150 Baronne Street, 907 Pierre Marquette Bldg., New Orleans 70112, (504) 568-5464

Executive Director, Louisiana State Board of Practical Nurse Examiners, 1440 Canal Street, Suite 2010, New Orleans 70012, (504) 568-6480

Maine

Executive Director, Maine State Board of Nursing, 295 Water Street, Augusta 04330, (207) 289-5324

Maryland

Executive Director, Maryland Board of Nurses, 4201 Patterson Avenue, Baltimore 21215, (301) 764-4747

Massachusetts

Executive Director, Massachusetts Board of Registration in Nursing, Everett Saltonstall Bldg., 100 Cambridge Street, Room 1519, Boston 02202, (617) 727-7393

Michigan

Administrative Assistant, Michigan Board of Nursing, Ottawa Towers North, 611 West Ottawa, P.O. Box 30018, Lansing 48909, (517) 373-1600

Minnesota

Executive Secretary, Minnesota Board of Nursing, 2700 University Ave. W., #108, St. Paul 55114, (612) 642-0567

Mississippi

Executive Director, Mississippi Board of Nursing, 239 North Lamar Street, Suite 401, Jackson 39201-1311, (601) 359-6170

Missouri

Executive Director, Missouri State Board of Nursing, P.O. Box 656, 3524 A North Ten Mile Drive, Jefferson City 65102, (314) 751-2334

Montana

Executive Secretary, Montana State Board of
Nursing, 1424 9th Avenue, Helena
59620-0407, (406) 444-4279

Nebraska

Nursing Licensure Coordinator, Bureau of
Examining Boards, Nebraska Department of
Health, P.O. Box 95007, Lincoln 68509,
(402) 471-2001

Nevada

Executive Secretary, Nevada State Board of
Nursing, 1281 Terminal Way, Suite 116, Reno
89502, (702) 786-2778

New Hampshire

Executive Director, New Hampshire Board of
Nursing, Health and Welfare Bldg., 6 Hazen
Dr., Concord 03301-6527, (603) 271-2323

New Jersey

Executive Director, New Jersey Board of Nursing,
1100 Raymond Blvd., Room 508, Newark
07102, (201) 648-2570

New Mexico

Executive Director, New Mexico Board of
Nursing, 4253 Montgomery N.E., Suite 130,
Albuquerque 87109, (505) 841-8340

New York

Executive Secretary, State Board of Nursing, State
Education Department, Cultural Education
Center, Rm. 9B30, Albany 12230,
(518) 474-3843/3844/3845

For licensing information

Supervisor, Division of Professional Licensing
Services, State Education Department, Cultural
Education Center, Albany 12230,
(518) 474-3817

North Carolina

Executive Director, North Carolina Board of
Nursing, P.O. Box 2129, Raleigh 27602,
(919) 782-3211

North Dakota

Executive Director, North Dakota Board for
Nursing, 919 South 7th St., Suite 504,
Bismarck 58504, (701) 224-2974

Ohio

Executive Secretary, Board of Nursing Education
and Nursing Registration, 77 S. High St., 17th
Floor, Columbus 43266-0316, (614) 466-3947

Oklahoma

Executive Director, Oklahoma Board of Nurse
Registration and Nursing Education, 2915 N.
Classen Blvd., Suite 524, Oklahoma City 73106,
(405) 525-2076

Oregon

Executive Director, Oregon State Board of
Nursing, 1400 S.W. 5th Avenue, Room 904,
Portland 97201, (503) 229-5653

Pennsylvania

Secretary, State Board of Nursing, P.O. Box 2649,
Harrisburg 17105-2649, (717) 783-7146

Puerto Rico

Puerto Rico Board of Nurse Examiners, 800
Roberto H. Todd Ave., Stop 18, Santurce
00908

Rhode Island

Executive Secretary, Rhode Island Board of Nurse
Registration and Nursing Education, Health
Department Building, 3 Capitol Hill, Room
104, Providence 02908-2488, (401) 277-2827

South Carolina

Executive Director, South Carolina State Board of
Nursing, 1777 St. Julian Place, Suite 102,
Columbia 29204, (803) 737-6594

South Dakota

Executive Secretary, South Dakota Board of
Nursing, 304 S. Phillips Avenue, Suite 205,
Sioux Falls 57102, (605) 335-4973

Tennessee

Executive Director, Tennessee State Board of
Nursing, 283 Plus Park Blvd., Nashville 37217,
(615) 367-6232

Texas

Executive Secretary, Board of Nurse Examiners
for Registered Nurses, 9100 Burnet Rd., Suite
104, Austin 78758, (512) 835-4880

Executive Director, Texas Board of Vocational
Nurse Examiners, 9100 Burnet Rd., Suite 105,
Austin 78758, (512) 835-2071

Utah

Executive Secretary, Utah State Board of Nursing, Division of Professional Licensing, Heber M. Wells Building, 160 East 300 South, P.O. Box 45802, Salt Lake City 84145, (801) 530-6628

Vermont

Executive Director, Vermont State Board of Nursing, Redstone Building, 26 Terrace St., Montpelier 05602, (802) 828-2396

Virginia

Executive Secretary, Virginia State Board of Nursing, 1601 Rolling Hills Dr., Richmond 23229-5005, (804) 662-9909

Virgin Islands

Executive Secretary, The Virgin Islands Board of Nurse Licensure, P.O. Box 7309, St. Thomas 00801, (809) 774-9000 Ext. 132

Washington

Executive Secretary, Washington State Board of Nursing, Division of Professional Licensing, P.O. Box 9649, Olympia 98504, (206) 753-3726

Executive Secretary, Washington State Board of Practical Nursing, P.O. Box 9649, Olympia 98504, (206) 586-1923

West Virginia

Executive Secretary, West Virginia Board of Examiners for Registered Nurses, 922 Quarrier Street, Suite 309, Embleton Building, Charleston 25301, (304) 348-3596

Executive Secretary, West Virginia State Board of Examiners for Practical Nurses, 922 Quarrier Street, Suite 506, Embleton Building, Charleston 25301, (304) 348-3572

Wisconsin

Director, Department of Regulation and Licensing, Bureau of Health Service Professions, Board of Nursing, P.O. Box 8935, Madison 53708-8935, (608) 266-3735

Wyoming

Executive Director, Wyoming State Board of Nursing, Barrett Bldg., 4th Floor, Cheyenne 82002, (307) 777-7601

Index